WORKBOOK TO ACCOMPANY
Mosby's EMT–Basic Textbook

Walt A. Stoy, PhD
and the
Center for Emergency Medicine

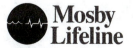

Mosby
Lifeline

St. Louis   Baltimore   Boston   Carlsbad   Chicago   Naples   New York   Philadelphia   Portland
London   Madrid   Mexico City   Singapore   Sydney   Tokyo   Toronto   Wiesbaden

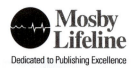

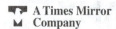

Dedicated to Publishing Excellence

A Times Mirror
Company

Senior Vice President: David T. Culverwell
Publisher: David Dusthimer
Executive Editor: Claire Merrick
Editor: Rina Steinhauer
Assistant Editor: Carla Goldberg
Project Manager: Chris Baumle
Production Editor: Anthony Trioli
Manufacturing Supervisor: William Winneberger

Printed in the United States of America
Composition by Shepherd, Inc.

Mosby–Year Book, Inc.
11830 Westline Industrial Drive
St. Louis, Missouri 63146

ISBN 0-8151-7959-6

PREFACE

This workbook is designed to accompany Mosby's EMT–Basic Textbook. Many students find it helpful to use a workbook to enhance their knowledge and retention after reading a textbook chapter. The goal of this workbook is to provide you with questions in various testing formats that will challenge you to think and analyze the possible alternatives in providing care to your patient.

Some students will elect to study by themselves, while others will benefit more by working with groups of students to complete the materials. Pairs or small study groups may use this workbook to challenge each other's knowledge about the material in each chapter. You may want to complete some portions of the text alone and use the examinations at the end of each division with groups of fellow students.

Your instructor may ask you to complete certain sections of the workbook as classroom assignments. This is an excellent way to test your knowledge of the material that is being presented.

There are two categories of questions found in this workbook - recall and recognition. Questions of recognition are true/false, matching and multiple choice. Recognition questions are designed to allow you to see the correct answer with distracting answers.

Questions of recall are completion, short answer and fill in the blank. These types of questions require you to know the answer. These are higher end educational questions that truly challenge your knowledge. This workbook has provided both recall and recognition questions for your educational enhancement.

Case studies are also included, that allow you to integrate knowledge from the current chapter and previous chapters to make patient care decisions.

The workbook chapters correspond to the chapters of the textbook. The following elements are found in most workbook chapters:

- Textbook chapter outline to facilitate note taking
- Key Term Matching exercise
- True or false questions
- Short answer/fill in the blank questions
- Multiple choice questions
- Case studies

Multiple choice examinations are provided at the end of each division to simulate exams you may take for certification.

In Section II of this workbook, you will find the answers to each question with a rationale explaining the critical points of knowledge. Each question is referenced to Mosby's EMT–Basic Textbook and to an objective from the EMT–Basic: National Standard Curriculum.

ACKNOWLEDGMENTS

Special thanks for much of the writing of this workbook to Elizabeth Criss, RN, and the staff of the Office of Education at the Center for Emergency Medicine.

PUBLISHER'S ACKNOWLEDGMENTS

The editors wish to acknowledge and thank the reviewers of this workbook, who devoted countless hours to intensive review. Their comments were invaluable in helping develop and fine tune this manuscript.

Barbara Aehlert, RN
Director, EMS Education and Research
Samaritan Health System
Phoenix, Arizona

Megan Archer, RN, BSN, CEN, MICN, NREMT-P
Education Coordinator
Emergency Department
Carolinas Medical Center
Charlotte, North Carolina

Chip Boehm, RN, EMT-P
Falmouth, Maine

Mick J. Sanders, EMT-P, MSA
St. Charles, Missouri

CONTENTS

QUESTIONS

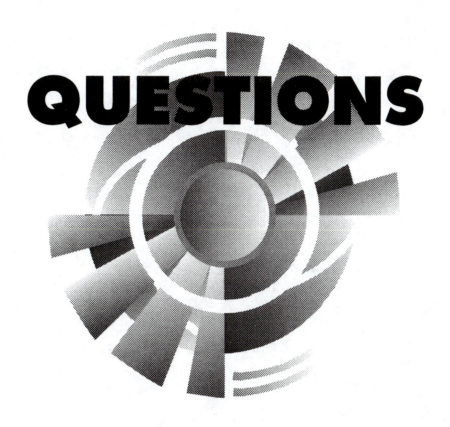

DIVISION ONE
PREPARATORY

CHAPTER 1

INTRODUCTION TO EMERGENCY MEDICAL CARE

● **CHAPTER OUTLINE**

I. The Emergency Medical Services System

    A. National Highway Traffic Safety Administration Technical Assistance Program

    B. Access to the Emergency Medical Services System

    C. Levels of Education

    D. The Healthcare System

    E. Liaison With Other Public Safety Workers

II. The Emergency Medical Technician-Basic

    A. Roles and Responsibilities

        1. Personal safety

        2. Safety of the crew, patient, and bystanders

        3. Patient assessment and care

        4. Lifting and moving patients

        5. Transport and transfer of care

        6. Patient advocacy

    B. Professional Attributes

III. Quality Care

    A. Quality Improvement

    B. Medical Direction

● MATCHING

Match the terms in Column 1 with the correct definition in Column 2:

Column 1

1. _____ Direct medical direction
2. _____ Emergency medical dispatcher
3. _____ EMS system
4. _____ Emergency Medical Technician
5. _____ EMT–Basic
6. _____ EMT–Intermediate
7. _____ EMT–Paramedic
8. _____ First Responder
9. _____ Indirect medical direction
10. _____ Medical direction
11. _____ National EMS Education and Practice Blueprint
12. _____ Quality improvement

Column 2

a. a method for planning, providing, and monitoring emergency care
b. the process of ensuring that care is medically appropriate
c. a method for evaluating and improving care
d. off-line activities like system design, education, and quality improvement
e. general term for a prehospital care provider
f. physicians speaking directly with personnel in the field
g. gives instructions over the phone until EMS arrives
h. highest level of EMT, with full advanced life-support capabilities
i. core content for scope of practice for EMS providers
j. provides initial emergency care until the ambulance arrives
k. EMTs with additional education such as vascular access, but not full advanced life support
l. EMT who provides primary care before the patient reaches the hospital

● REVIEW QUESTIONS

1. Communications and universal access are part of the National Highway Traffic Safety Administration's (NHTSA) 10 standards for EMS. **True or false?**
2. NHTSA's facilities standard helps ensure that patients are transported to the closest appropriate hospital. **True or false?**
3. The role of a First Responder is to:
   a. Stabilize and transport an ill or injured person
   b. Provide advanced care to an ill or injured person
   c. Provide advanced care without transporting an ill or injured person
   d. Provide initial stabilization until more advanced EMS personnel arrive
4. The EMT–Basic course prepares people to:
   a. Provide advanced care for trauma patients
   b. Start an IV and administer medications
   c. Manage life-threatening illnesses and injuries
   d. Stabilize a patient's injury until further help arrives
5. List three ways to help ensure personal safety:

   a. _____

   b. _____

   c. _____

6. EMT–Basics are responsible for the safety of their crew and the patient, and police and other emergency workers are responsible for the safety of bystanders. **True or false?**

7. List three roles and responsibilities of the EMT–Basic:

   a. _____

   b. _____

   c. _____

8. Which of the following characteristics of the EMT may help reduce patient and family anxiety:
   a. Professional manner
   b. Confident attitude
   c. Clean, tidy uniform
   d. All of the above

9. Which term is used to describe the physician who monitors the activities of an EMS system:
   a. Physician in charge
   b. Trauma physician
   c. Medical director
   d. EMS physician

10. Direct medical direction and on-line medical direction refer to face-to-face, telephone, or radio communication between the physician and EMS provider. **True or false?**

11. Define quality improvement:

   _____

   _____

   _____

12. Which of the following best defines medical direction?
   a. Can be on-line or off-line
   b. Can have protocols or standing orders
   c. Physician's monitoring of the care of EMT–Basics
   d. All of the above

13. You have been asked to speak at an elementary school during Health Awareness Week. The school principal wants you to describe your job and to explain how students can access healthcare during an emergency.
   a. What are the roles and responsibilities of the EMT–Basic?

   _____

   _____

   b. What are the components that encompass an EMS response?

   _____

   _____

   c. How can citizens access the EMS system?

   _____

   _____

CHAPTER 2
THE WELL-BEING OF THE EMT-BASIC

● CHAPTER OUTLINE

I. Emotional Aspects of Emergency Care

    A. Death and Dying

    B. Stressful Situations

    C. Stress Management

    D. Critical Incident Stress Debriefing

    E. Comprehensive Critical Incident Stress Management

II. Scene Safety

    A. Body Substance Isolation Precautions

        1. Hand washing

        2. Eye protection

        3. Gloves

        4. Gowns

        5. Masks

        6. Reporting an exposure

    B. Advance Safety Precautions

    C. Personal Protection

        1. Hazardous materials

        2. Rescue

        3. Violence

● MATCHING

Match the terms in Column 1 with the correct definition in Column 2:

	Column 1		Column 2
1. _____	BSI precautions	a.	tension resulting from physical, chemical, or emotional factors
2. _____	Critical incident	b.	causes unusually strong reactions and interferes with work
3. _____	Critical incident stress debriefing	c.	process to help emergency workers deal with emotions and feelings
4. _____	Hazardous material	d.	steps taken to prevent exposure to blood or other body fluids
5. _____	Stress	e.	substance that poses an unreasonable risk on release

6. Number the five stages in the death and dying process, with 1 as the first stage and 5 as the last:

_____ Anger   _____ Acceptance

_____ Bargaining   _____ Depression

_____ Denial

7. Indicate the order of the scene responsibilities of the EMT–Basic, with 1 as the first priority and 4 as the last:

_____ The patient's safety   _____ Bystander safety

_____ Personal safety   _____ Other crew members' safety

● REVIEW QUESTIONS

1. All people move through the stages of death and dying at the same rate. **True or false?**
2. List two actions the EMT–Basic may take to help the family members of a patient who is dying deal with their emotions:

   a. _____

   b. _____

3. Which of the following is a stress reduction technique?
   a. Quiting smoking
   b. Volunteering as an EMT–Basic somewhere outside of your job
   c. Decreasing exercise programs
   d. Maintaining a constant work schedule
4. EMT–Basics may experience emotions such as guilt and anxiety, even when they have treated a patient to the best of their abilities. **True or false?**
5. List three situations that may cause stress for the EMT–Basic:

   a. _____

   b. _____

   c. _____

6. Stress can be caused by _____,

_____, or _____ factors.

7. List three warning signs of stress:

a. _____

b. _____

c. _____

8. A critical level of stress can be the result of one incident or a slow build-up over time. **True or false?**

9. The purpose of Critical Incident Stress Debriefing is to help the EMT–Basic speed up the normal recovery process. **True or false?**

10. Families of EMT–Basics seldom face stresses related to their outside involvement in the profession of EMS. **True or false?**

11. EMT–Basics are experiencing critical incident stress when:

a. Their emotional reactions interfere with their ability to function

b. They feel guilty about the death of a patient

c. They doubt that they treated a patient appropriately

d. They are unable to relate their feelings to their family

12. EMT–Basics should determine scene safety immediately after assessing the patient's airway, breathing, and circulation. **True or false?**

13. Which of the following combinations of body substance isolation precautions should be worn when caring for an injury with minimal bleeding?

a. Gloves only   c. Gloves and mask

b. Gloves, protective eyewear   d. Mask only

14. Eye protection and masks should be worn when there is a possibility that blood or body fluids could splash during patient care. **True or false?**

15. EMT–Basics responding to a hazardous materials incident should _____.

a. Assume command of the scene

b. Begin treatment and transport of all ill or injured persons

c. Wait until a specialized hazardous materials team secures the scene

d. None of the above

16. Turn-out gear, puncture-proof gloves, steel-toed boots, and a helmet are the type of equipment necessary for _____.

a. Most hazardous materials   c. Routine emergencies

b. Most rescue situations   d. Firefighting only

17. You have been dispatched to the home of a terminally ill patient who has been involved in a hospice program. The patient's wife is distraught, and her daughter has requested EMS assistance.

a. Describe, in order, the stages most patients and family members go through when they discover that death is imminent.

_____

_____

b. When you arrive at the scene, the wife pleads with you to "please do something to make him live another day." This is an example of which stage?

_____

_____

c. How should you deal with the family members in this situation?

_____

_____

18. Over the past several weeks, your partner has been a little hard to get along with. She has been very quiet and withdrawn and does not talk much to anybody.
    a. You know that your partner is showing warning signs of stress. What are other stress warning signs?

_____

_____

    b. List seven techniques that can reduce stress and help to avoid burnout.

_____

_____

    c. Describe situations that can cause stress in EMS.

_____

_____

CHAPTER 3

MEDICAL/LEGAL AND ETHICAL ISSUES

● **CHAPTER OUTLINE**

    I. Scope of Practice

       A. Legal Duties to the Patient, Medical Director, and Public

       B. Ethical Responsibilities

       C. Duty to Act

          1. Legal considerations

             a. Negligence

             b. Abandonment

          2. Ethical considerations

   II. Consent for Treatment and Transport

       A. Expressed Consent

       B. Implied Consent

       C. Children and Mentally Incompetent Adults

       D. Refusal of Treatment and Transport

       E. Assault and Battery

       F. Advance Directives

          1. Living wills

          2. Durable Power of Attorney

          3. Do Not Resuscitate orders

  III. Patient Confidentiality

       A. Confidential Information

       B. Releasing Confidential Information

       C. Situations Requiring Special Reporting

  IV. Special Situations

       A. Potential Organ Donors

       B. Medical Condition Identification Insignia

       C. Considerations at Possible Crime Scenes

● MATCHING

Match the terms in Column 1 with the correct definition in Column 2:

Column 1

1. _____ Abandonment

2. _____ Advance directives

3. _____ Assault

4. _____ Battery

5. _____ Duty to act

6. _____ Expressed consent

7. _____ Implied consent

8. _____ Negligence

9. _____ Scope of practice

10. _____ Standard of care

Column 2

a. minimum acceptable level of treatment within a community

b. duties and skills that can be performed by an EMT–Basic

c. failure to act in a reasonable and prudent manner

d. condition to provide care when a patient is physically, mentally, or emotionally unable to consent

e. legal obligation to provide care when opportunity exists

f. condition in which the patient agrees and gives permission for treatment

g. termination of care without consent or transfer to an equal or higher level of provider

h. threatening or attempting to inflict offensive physical contact

i. orders regarding care to be given in certain emergency situations

j. offensive touching of a person without his/her consent

● REVIEW QUESTIONS

1. In most states, the EMT–Basic's scope of practice is based on which of the following?
   a. The US Department of Transportation National Highway Safety Administration's National Standard Curriculum
   b. The individual medical director for each agency
   c. Each individual EMT–Basic
   d. The service or agency to which the EMT–Basic belongs

2. Protocols and standing orders are used to narrow the scope of practice for EMT-Basics. **True or false?**

3. What conditions would cause an EMT–Basic to have a "duty to act"?

_____

_____

_____

4. List the four criteria necessary for an EMT-Basic to be accused of negligence:

   a. _____

   b. _____

   c. _____

   d. _____

5. In which of these situations can you release the patient for continued care and not be accused of abandonment?
   a. EMT–Basic to a bystander
   c. EMT–Basic to First Responder
   b. EMT–Basic to the hospital staff
   d. EMT–Paramedic to EMT-Basic
6. The term that describes permission to be treated is called

   _____.
7. Children have the right to refuse care, even if their parents consent for them to be treated. **True or false?**
8. What steps should the EMT–Basic take when a patient refuses treatment or transport?

   _____

   _____

   _____

9. Threatening to touch someone without his/her permission is called:
   a. Aggression
   c. Assault
   b. Battery
   d. Negligence
10. Advance directives are written documents used to express patients' wishes for the type of care they want or do not want in the future. **True or false?**
11. List three situations when an EMT–Basic can release confidential information:

    a. _____

    b. _____

    c. _____
12. Which of the following is **NOT** a reportable case in most states?
    a. Gunshot wounds
    c. Motor vehicle crashes
    b. Child or elder abuse
    d. Animal bites
13. Patients who are dying can become organ donors by making their wishes known to an EMT–Basic when they are dying. **True or false?**
14. When treating a victim of a violent crime, the EMT–Basic should never disturb the crime scene. **True or false?**
15. Last year, you worked a call involving a motor vehicle crash. There were two patients with serious injuries and one fatality. One of the survivors now claims that you did not perform to the standard of care and were negligent in your delivery of emergency care.
    a. Define standard of care.

    _____

    _____

    b. Define negligence.

    _____

    _____

    c. List the four criteria that must be met before negligence can be proven.

    _____

    _____

16. You are caring for a patient who has fallen and struck his head. He is unresponsive and has a notable amount of bleeding from a scalp laceration.
    a. How would you obtain permission to treat this patient?

_____

    b. What is the legal basis that allows you to initiate emergency care?

_____

    c. Define expressed consent.

_____

17. You are caring for a 68-year-old man who collapsed at his neighbor's home from cardiac arrest. The automated external defibrillator is applied, CPR is in progress, and the patient is intubated. The patient's son arrives on the scene and advises you that he has Durable Power of Attorney for his father's healthcare. His father is terminally ill and has signed a living will that requests he not be resuscitated. He demands that you stop CPR and allow his father to "die in peace."
    a. What is a living will?

_____

    b. What is Durable Power of Attorney?

_____

    c. How will you handle this situation?

_____

_____

CHAPTER 4
THE HUMAN BODY

● **CHAPTER OUTLINE**

I. Anatomic Terms

    A. The Anatomic Position

    B. Descriptive Anatomic Terms

II. Body Systems

    A. The Respiratory System

        1. The airway

        2. The lungs

            a. Gas exchange

        3. Normal breathing

        4. The respiratory system of infants and children

    B. The Circulatory System

        1. The heart

        2. Blood vessels

        3. The blood

        4. The circulation of blood

    C. The Musculoskeletal System

        1. The skeleton

            a. The skull

            b. The spinal column and rib cage

            c. The pelvis and lower extremities

            d. The upper extremities

        2. Joints

        3. Muscles

            a. Skeletal muscles

            b. Smooth muscles

            c. Cardiac muscles

    D. The Nervous System

    E. The Skin

    F. The Digestive System

    G. The Endocrine System

● MATCHING

Match the terms in Column 1 with the correct definition in Column 2:

Column 1	Column 2
1. _____ Accessory breathing muscles	a. a measure of the force exerted against the arterial walls
2. _____ Adrenaline	b. number of heart beats in 1 minute
3. _____ Anatomic position	c. standing upright with feet, palms, eyes facing forward
4. _____ Bilateral	d. a pulse point in an extremity
5. _____ Blood pressure	e. body defense against infection
6. _____ Breath sounds	f. sound made by air moving in and out of the lungs
7. _____ Central pulse	g. a pulse point in or near the trunk
8. _____ Heart rate	h. used in respiratory distress to draw more air into the lungs
9. _____ Hemoglobin	i. regulate body activities and functions in many body systems
10. _____ Hormones	j. the volume of air per breath
11. _____ Insulin	k. the process of circulating blood, delivering oxygen, and removing waste
12. _____ Intercostal muscles	l. line from the armpits to the ankles, dividing the body in halves
13. _____ Midaxillary line	m. the right and left sides of the body relative to each other
14. _____ Midclavicular line	n. a hormone that helps prepare the body for emergencies
15. _____ Midline	o. bone structure composed of 12 pairs of ribs and the sternum
16. _____ Perfusion	p. line through the middle of the body through nose and umbilicus
17. _____ Peripheral pulse	q. blood cells containing hemoglobin
18. _____ Platelets	r. two lines dividing the collar bone in two, extending through the nipples
19. _____ Red blood cells	s. blood component that plays a role in clotting
20. _____ Sutures	t. carries oxygen in blood and releases it when it reaches the tissue
21. _____ Thorax	u. hormone crucial for the body's use of sugar
22. _____ Tidal volume	v. muscles between each rib that move with breathing
23. _____ White blood cells	w. joints between the skull bones

24. Label Figure 4-1 with the following directional terms:

anterior   lateral
medial   inferior
midaxillary line midline
posterior   superior

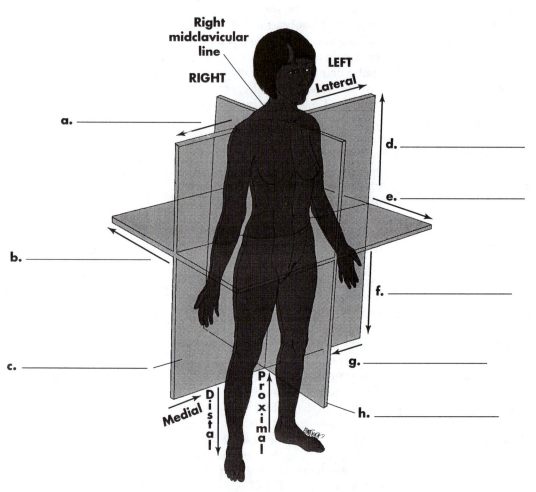

Figure 4-1

25. Label Figure 4-2 with the following skeletal structures:

vertebral column   mandible
femur   sternum
ribs   patella
clavicle   pelvis
skull   tibia
humerus   radius

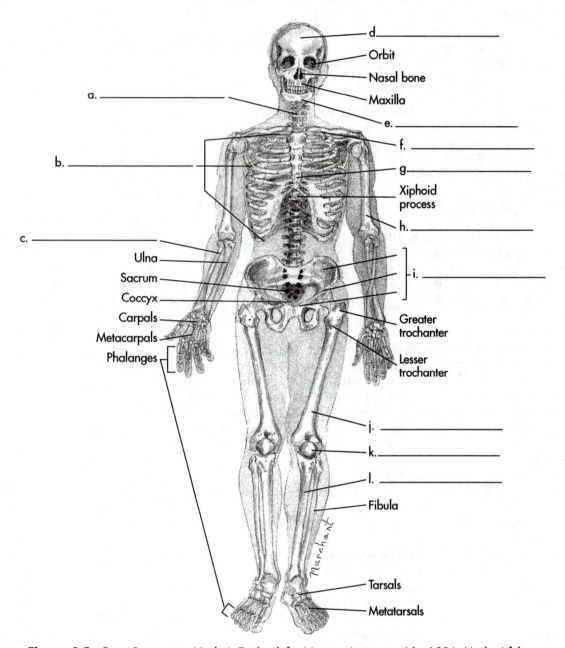

Figure 4-2   From Sorrentino: *Mosby's Textbook for Nursing Assistants,* 4/e, 1996, Mosby Lifeline.

● REVIEW QUESTIONS

1. The midaxillary line divides the body into the _____

   and _____ planes.
   - **a.** Anterior; posterior
   - **c.** Posterior; medial
   - **b.** Superior; inferior
   - **d.** Anterior; inferior

2. Which of the following terms is used to describe the portion of the throat directly behind the mouth?
   - **a.** Nasopharynx
   - **c.** Larynx
   - **b.** Epiglottis
   - **d.** Oropharynx

3. The trachea is the anatomic term for the _____.
   - **a.** Windpipe
   - **c.** Lungs
   - **b.** Throat
   - **d.** Mouth

4. The two main sets of muscles used during the normal breathing process are the _____ and the _____.
   - **a.** Diaphragm; intervertebral muscles
   - **b.** Intercostal muscles; bronchi
   - **c.** Diaphragm; intercostal muscles
   - **d.** None of the above

5. Which of the following best describes the action of the diaphragm during inspiration?
   - **a.** The muscle fibers relax, the dome flattens and lowers
   - **b.** The muscle fibers contract, the dome flattens and lowers
   - **c.** The muscle fibers relax, the dome flattens and raises
   - **d.** The muscle fibers contract, the dome flattens and raises

6. The heart is a pump and consists of _____ chambers.
   - **a.** 2
   - **c.** 6
   - **b.** 4
   - **d.** 8

7. Which of the following best describes the flow of blood through the heart?
   - **a.** Right ventricle, right atrium, lungs, left atrium, left ventricle, body
   - **b.** Right atrium, right ventricle, lungs, left atrium, left ventricle, body
   - **c.** Left atrium, left ventricle, lungs, right atrium, right ventricle, body
   - **d.** Right ventricle, right atrium, lungs, left ventricle, left atrium, body

8. _____ carry the blood away from the heart, _____ carry blood to the heart.
   - **a.** Veins; arteries
   - **c.** Arteries; capillaries
   - **b.** Veins; capillaries
   - **d.** Arteries; veins

9. How many liters of blood does the average-sized adult man have in his body?
   - **a.** 3-4
   - **c.** 2-4
   - **b.** 5-6
   - **d.** 7-8

10. The first number recorded in the blood pressure is the _____.
    - **a.** Systolic pressure
    - **c.** Aortic pressure
    - **b.** Diastolic pressure
    - **d.** Venous pressure

11. Match the muscles in Column 1 to their location in Column 2:

Column 1	Column 2
_____ Smooth muscle	**a.** located in the heart
	b. located in the stomach and intestines
_____ Skeletal muscle	
	c. attaches to bones
_____ Cardiac muscle	

12. The central nervous system consists of _____.
    a. The brain and spinal cord
    b. The brain and the peripheral nerves
    c. The spinal cord and peripheral nerves
    d. The brain and sensory nerves
13. The peripheral nerves carry information between the spinal column and the other parts of the body. **True or false?**
14. Signals from the motor nerves cause contractions in the skeletal muscles. **True or false?**
15. The skin has _____ layers.
    a. 3   c. 2
    b. 4   d. 1
16. What is the role of the digestive system?

_____

_____

17. Chemicals released from glands within the body are called

_____.

18. You are observing an autopsy as part of a continuing education program. After exposing the thoracic cavity, the medical examiner performing the autopsy asks you the following questions:
    a. Where do the bronchi begin and end?

_____

_____

    b. What muscles are involved in the process of ventilation and how do they work during inhalation and exhalation?

_____

_____

    c. How does gas exchange occur in the alveoli?

_____

_____

_____

19. You are working at a local health fair to assist with blood pressure screenings. A middle-aged woman asks you to take her blood pressure and explain to her the meaning of the two numbers in the measurement. The reading you obtain is 184/96.
    a. How would you explain blood pressure measurement to her?

_____

_____

_____

b. How would you explain the meaning of the two measurement numbers?

_____

_____

_____

c. What else should you tell this woman about her blood pressure reading?

_____

_____

_____

20. You are hosting an EMT–Basic study group for your classmates at your home. The group decides to take a break from studying and to play "EMS Jeopardy." What are the questions to the answers provided below?
   a. They are muscles that are attached to bones.

   _____

   b. This system consists of sensory and motor nerves that lie outside the skull or spinal cord.

   _____

   c. It is the layer of skin that contains sweat glands, hair follicles, blood vessels, and nerve endings.

   _____

CHAPTER 5
BASELINE VITAL SIGNS AND SAMPLE HISTORY

● **CHAPTER OUTLINE**

I. Baseline Vital Signs

    A. Breathing

        1. Rate

        2. Quality

    B. Pulse

        1. Rate

        2. Quality

    C. Skin

        1. Color

        2. Temperature

        3. Condition

        4. Capillary refill

    D. Pupils

    E. Blood Pressure

    F. Vital Sign Reassessment

II. SAMPLE History

● MATCHING

Match the terms in Column 1 with the correct definition in Column 2:

Column 1	Column 2
1. _____ Accessory muscle	a. an increase in the effort expended to breathe
2. _____ Capillary refill	b. amount of time required for blood to return to vessels after applying pressure
3. _____ Crowing	c. a long, high-pitched sound when breathing in
4. _____ Diastolic blood pressure	d. high-pitched whistling sound caused by constriction of the smaller airways
5. _____ Grunting	e. referring to pupil constriction when exposed to light
6. _____ Gurgling	f. a condition that can be observed and identified in the patient
7. _____ History	g. additional muscles used to breathe by patients in respiratory distress
8. _____ Labored respirations	h. sound made because of the tongue falling back and partially obstructing the airway
9. _____ Noisy respirations	i. sound made when exhaling forcefully against a closed glottis
10. _____ Normal respirations	j. measurement of pressure against the arteries when the heart contracts
11. _____ Reactive to light	k. a nonobservable condition described by the patient
12. _____ Shallow respirations	l. a loud, high-pitched airway noise that usually occurs during inspiration, can indicate obstruction
13. _____ Sign	m. comparing sets of vital signs over time
14. _____ Snoring	n. any sound coming from the patient's airway; indicates a problem
15. _____ Stridor	o. low volumes of air on inspiration and expiration
16. _____ Symptom	p. respirations without noise or effort; occur at a rate of 12-20 per minute in adult patients
17. _____ Systolic blood pressure	q. a concise and inclusive set of information the EMT–Basic gathers about the patient
18. _____ Trending	r. measurement of pressure against the arteries when the heart is at rest
19. _____ Wheezing	s. sound made when there is liquid in the airway

● REVIEW QUESTIONS

1. When assessing breathing, assess the rate and _____ of the respirations.
2. The average respiratory rate for an adult at rest is _____.
   - a. 10-15
   - b. 12-26
   - c. 10-20
   - d. 12-20

3. How would you assess a patient's respiratory rate?

_____

_____

4. The noise made by the tongue partially blocking the airway is called crowing. **True or false?**
5. The pulse can be felt where a vein passes over a bone near the surface of the skin. **True or false?**
6. When assessing a patient's pulse, note the _____ (by

   counting the number of beats in _____ seconds and

   multiplying by 2), and _____.
7. The average resting pulse rate for an adult should be _____.
   a. 60-80   **c.** 60-100
   b. 50-100   **d.** 50-80
8. Define the following terms:

   Regular pulse- _____

   Irregular pulse- _____

   Weak pulse- _____
9. Which of the following are the components of the assessment of the skin?
   a. Quality, color, and motor function
   b. Temperature and motor and sensory function
   c. Color, temperature, and condition
   d. None of the above
10. When assessing skin color in the nail beds, oral mucosa, or conjunctive, the normal skin color is pink, and abnormal skin colors include

    _____ or red, cyanotic or _____,

    _____ or yellow, and pale.

11. To identify skin temperature, the skin of the _____ is more reliable than the skin of the extremities.
12. List three abnormal skin temperatures and the conditions that may cause them:

    a. _____

    b. _____

    c. _____
13. The normal skin condition is _____, and abnormal skin conditions include _____, _____, and _____ skin.
    a. moist; dry, wet, cracked
    b. dry; moist, wet, extremely dry
    c. dry; extremely dry, yellow, moist
    d. moist; wet, extremely dry, and cold
14. Normal capillary refill in an infant or child should take less than _____ seconds.
    a. 1   **c.** 3
    b. 2   **d.** 4

15. _____ pupils are big and _____ pupils are small.

16. Define the terms *equal* and *reactive to light* in relation to the pupil of the eye.

_____

_____

_____

17. When pupils react normally to light, they _____.
    a. Dilate   c. Constrict
    b. Remain unchanged   d. One constricts, one dilates

18. How would you assess a patient's pupils in bright sunlight?

_____

_____

19. Blood pressure is a measure of the amount of force exerted on the blood vessel walls during each heart beat. **True or false?**

20. Blood pressure can be measured by listening with a stethoscope, called

_____, or by feeling for the return of a pulse, called

_____.

21. Reassess stable patients every _____ minutes and unstable patients every _____ minutes.
    a. 5; 15   c. 15; 10
    b. 6; 10   d. 15; 5

22. The 'A' in the SAMPLE history stands for allergies. **True or false?**

23. Past medical history should include a detailed account of any medical condition the patient may have experienced. **True or false?**

24. Medical identification tags generally do not provide any information that is pertinent in the prehospital setting. **True or false?**

25. List two reasons why it is important to accurately record a patient's history and vital signs:

    a. _____

    b. _____

26. You are participating in a clinical rotation at a local pediatrician's office. You have been asked to take a complete set of vital signs on three patients.
    a. What is a normal respiratory rate range for a 1-year-old child?

    _____

    b. What is a normal pulse rate range for a 3-year-old child?

    _____

    c. What is a normal blood pressure range for a 7-year-old child?

    _____

27. You have been dispatched to care for a patient with difficulty breathing. On arrival, you find a 28-year-old man with labored respirations and audible wheezing. His wife tells you that he has a history of asthma.
  a. What two components do you evaluate in a respiratory assessment?

  _____

  _____

  b. If the patient is in respiratory distress, what accessory muscles might he use to assist with breathing?

  _____

  _____

  c. How would you describe "wheezing"?

  _____

  _____

CHAPTER 6
LIFTING AND MOVING PATIENTS

● **CHAPTER OUTLINE**

I. Body Mechanics

    A. Lifting

    B. Carrying

    C. Reaching

    D. Pushing and Pulling

II. Principles of Moving Patients

    A. Emergency Moves

    B. Urgent Moves

    C. Nonurgent Moves

III. Equipment

    A. Stretchers and Cots

        1. Wheeled stretcher

        2. Portable stretcher

        3. Scoop stretcher

        4. Flexible stretcher

        5. Basket stretcher

        6. Stair chair

        7. Backboards

    B. Patient Positioning

● MATCHING

Match the terms in Column 1 with the correct definition in Column 2:

Column 1	Column 2
1. _____ Body mechanics	**a.** a move required when there is danger to the crew or patient if the patient is not moved
2. _____ Emergency move	**b.** left-lateral recumbent position, used for unresponsive, nontrauma patients
3. _____ Nonurgent move	**c.** a move used when there are no immediate threats
4. _____ Power grip	**d.** principles of movement used during lifting and moving
5. _____ Recovery position	**e.** a patient move used when the patient's condition may become life threatening
6. _____ Urgent move	**f.** hand position providing maximum force to the object being lifted

● REVIEW QUESTIONS

1. You and your partner should be able and prepared to lift and move every patient for whom you care. **True or false?**
2. List two components of safe lifting or carrying:

   a. _____

   b. _____
3. Carrying a patient should always be avoided. **True or false?**
4. One-handed carrying techniques are dangerous—EMTs should always use two hands when lifting. **True or false?**
5. What is the safest way to carry a patient down a flight of stairs?

   _____

   _____
6. Avoid lifting situations when you must reach more than _____ in front of you and when you must reach for more than _____.
   a. 20 inches; 30 seconds   c. 25 inches; 30 seconds
   b. 20 inches; 1 minute   d. 25 inches; 1 minute
7. Describe how to reach safely when performing a log roll.

   _____

   _____
8. It is always preferable to _____ rather than _____ any object.
   a. Push; pull   c. Carry; pull
   b. Pull; push   d. Push; drag
9. Although you will not take time to immobilize a patient during an emergency move, consideration should be given to protecting the _____.
10. If there is an immediate danger for the patient, such as fire, explosives, or other hazards, how should the patient be moved?
    a. Urgent move   c. Nonurgent move
    b. Emergency move   d. Rapid extrication move

11. Spinal stabilization techniques can be implemented with an urgent move. **True or false?**

12. Match the following pieces of equipment with the correct application:

_____ Long backboard   **a.** lift from a supine position to a stretcher

                                  b. immobilize an entire patient

_____ Scoop stretcher   **c.** move patient through narrow halls

                                  d. immobilization during extrication

_____ Stair chair   when the patient is in a seated position

                                  e. can be attached to ropes and other

_____ Basket stretcher   lifting devices for rescue situations

_____ Short backboard

13. When transporting a pregnant patient in the ambulance, she usually should be placed on her _____.
    a. Left side   **c.** Back
    b. Right side   **d.** Abdomen

14. An unresponsive patient with a suspected spinal injury should be placed in the recovery position. **True or false?**

15. How should a patient with signs and symptoms of shock (hypoperfusion) be transported?
    a. Flat on the back
    b. Head up 30 degrees
    c. Flat on the back, legs elevated 8 to 12 inches
    d. Head down 30°

16. How should a responsive patient who is nauseated or vomiting and has no suspected trauma be positioned for transport?
    a. In the position of comfort   **c.** On left side
    b. Supine   **d.** Head up 15°

17. You have been dispatched to a patient with a possible allergic reaction. When you arrive at the scene you are directed up a steep flight of stairs to the attic in an older home. There, you find a 56-year-old man who was replacing fiberglass insulation when he became short of breath. You apply high-concentration oxygen and assess his vital signs. He is responsive and alert but says he is too weak to walk down the steps.
    a. What would be the best method of moving this patient to the main level of the house?

    _____

    b. When would use of this moving device be contraindicated?

    _____

    c. If this patient had also fallen, how should he be transported?

    _____

    _____

18. You have responded to a motor vehicle crash where fire and rescue personnel are on the scene. On arrival, you find the driver of the car trapped behind the steering column. The fire department has provided access through the driver's door. The patient is unresponsive and has gurgling respirations and an open chest injury.

a. What are your first actions in providing care for this patient?

_____

_____

_____

b. Is this patient a candidate for rapid extrication? If so, why?

_____

_____

_____

c. Describe the general principles of rapid extrication.

_____

_____

_____

Directions: Circle the letter of the correct answer.

1. EMT–Basics are best defined as:
   a. Responders to stabilize the patient until advanced help arrives
   b. Definitive care for trauma patients
   c. Advanced level of prehospital care provider
   d. Providers of primary care before the patient reaches the hospital

2. Which of the following statements is true concerning EMS?
   a. EMT–Basics rarely interact with other public safety workers
   b. EMT–Basics should be concerned with the patient's rights
   c. EMT–Basics should put the needs of the patient first, before their personal safety
   d. EMT–Basics require little continuing education

3. Which of the following is **NOT** a role and responsibility of the EMT–Basic?
   a. Patient assessment   c. Transport and transfer of care
   b. Personal safety   d. Care based on diagnosis

4. The first priority of the EMT–Basic at the scene of an emergency should always be:
   a. Scene and personal safety
   b. Communication with the patient
   c. Correct documentation
   d. Contacting medical direction

5. Physician medical directors:
   a. Are not involved in postcall quality improvement
   b. Are rarely involved in the development of protocols
   c. Should be involved in the education of EMT–Basics
   d. Are not involved in patient care decisions at the scene

6. Which of the following is **NOT** a stage of death and dying?
   a. Anger   c. Bargaining
   b. Denial   d. Sympathy

7. Which of the following statements is true when dealing with the dying patient and family members?
   a. Patient needs include dignity, respect, sharing, communications, privacy, and control
   b. Separate the patient from the family members when possible
   c. Provide false reassurance if necessary to make the family feel better
   d. Do not touch the patient unless medically necessary

8. What is CISD?
   a. Critical Injury Stabilization Disorder
   b. Clinical Incident Stress Disorder
   c. Clinical Injury Situation Debriefing
   d. Critical Incident Stress Debriefing

9. Which of the following are components of CISD?
   a. Preincident stress education   c. Spouse and family support
   b. On-scene peer support   d. All of the above

10. Which of the following is associated with body substance isolation precautions?
    a. Industrial grade goggles
    b. Self-contained breathing apparatus
    c. Masks with eye shields
    d. Helmets with chin straps

11. Negligence occurs when:
    a. Continued care is not assured for a patient at the same or higher level
    b. A patient suffers damages or injury because an EMT–Basic fails to perform at the accepted level of care
    c. The EMT–Basic treats the patient without consent
    d. The EMT–Basic continues to treat the patient after he/she has refused treatment
12. Which of the following statements regarding consent is true?
    a. Expressed consent can be provided by responsive and unresponsive patients
    b. Use implied consent to treat the unresponsive patient
    c. Use implied consent to treat children whose parents do not want them to be treated
    d. The patient cannot withdraw his/her consent once it is given
13. Which of the following statements is true concerning refusals in patient care?
    a. Children can refuse care, even if their parents want them to be treated
    b. The patient cannot withdraw from treatment after it has begun
    c. Patients who do not want care must simply sign a release
    d. When in doubt if there is consent to treatment, err in the favor of treatment
14. Which of the following statements is true regarding Do Not Resuscitate (DNR) orders?
    a. The patient has the right to refuse certain resuscitation efforts
    b. In general, DNR orders don't require written orders from physicians
    c. All states recognize DNR orders for prehospital personnel
    d. The DNR order does not have to be seen by the EMT–Basic to be honored
15. In which of the following situations can an EMT–Basic release confidential information?
    a. In a case review for continuing education
    b. Any time law enforcement personnel request information
    c. When there is a reportable situation
    d. All of the above
16. Which of the following terms is associated with the respiratory system?
    a. Pharynx   c. Olecranon process
    b. Mitral valve   d. Adrenaline
17. Which of the following is true concerning anatomic considerations in infants and children?
    a. In general, all structures are smaller and less easily obstructed
    b. The tongue is smaller proportionally and rarely causes problems
    c. The trachea is more easily obstructed by swelling
    d. The trachea is less flexible because it is less developed
18. Which of the following statements about the circulatory system is true?
    a. Oxygenated blood is pumped from the lungs to the left atrium
    b. The average man has approximately 5 gallons of blood
    c. Platelets are important for fighting infection
    d. The upper chambers of the heart are the ventricles
19. What is the medical terminology used to describe the bone in the thigh?
    a. Tibia   c. Fibula
    b. Femur   d. Patella
20. Which of the following statements is true?
    a. The digestive system contains glands that release hormones
    b. The motor nerves carry information to the brain from the body
    c. The middle layer of the skin is the dermis
    d. The central nervous system is composed of motor and sensory nerves

21. The average pulse rate range for an adult is:
    a. 12-20   c. 70-100
    b. 60-80   d. 50-70
22. Which of the following is a characteristic of normal breathing?
    a. Increased effort   c. Using accessory muscles
    b. Grunting and stridor   d. Bilateral chest expansion
23. Which of the following terms is used to describe a patient's skin temperature?
    a. Hot   c. Clammy
    b. Dry   d. Pale
24. Which of the following statements is correct?
    a. Pupils should dilate equally when exposed to light
    b. Capillary refill should be assessed in patients less than 6 years of age
    c. The diastolic pressure is the measurement of force exerted when the heart is contracting
    d. Vital signs should be reassessed every 15 minutes for unstable patients
25. Which of the following statements concerning the SAMPLE history is correct?
    a. The "A" in SAMPLE stands for allergies to medications only
    b. A complete past medical history should be assessed
    c. A symptom is any medical condition that can be observed
    d. The "E" in SAMPLE stands for Events leading to the illness or injury
26. Which of the following statements is true concerning lifting and moving?
    a. Use legs, not back, to lift
    b. Use back, not legs, to lift
    c. Twist when needed to help move patients
    d. Use no more than three people to move a patient
27. Which of the following is a dangerous way to lift a stretcher?
    a. Using the power-lift
    b. Using the power-grip
    c. Bending at the waist
    d. Lifting while keeping back in locked-in position
28. Which of the following is true regarding moving patients?
    a. An emergency move is necessary if you cannot provide life-saving care because of the patient's position
    b. Use urgent moves when there is an immediate danger present
    c. There is no time for spinal protection during urgent moves
    d. A patient with signs and symptoms of shock would require a nonurgent move
29. How should the unresponsive patient, without suspected spine injury, be transported?
    a. In the recovery position   c. Prone
    b. Supine   d. In the position of comfort
30. How should a responsive patient with chest pain or difficulty breathing and no signs of trauma be transported?
    a. In the recovery position   c. Prone
    b. Supine   d. In the position of comfort

DIVISION TWO
AIRWAY

CHAPTER 7

THE AIRWAY

● **CHAPTER OUTLINE**

I. The Respiratory System

   A. Respiratory Anatomy

   B. Respiratory Physiology

      1. Adequate breathing

      2. Inadequate breathing

      3. Considerations for infants and children

II. Oxygen

   A. Oxygen Sources

   B. Equipment for Oxygen Delivery

      1. Oxygen regulators

      2. Masks

         a. Nonrebreather masks

         b. Nasal cannulas

III. Opening the Airway

   A. Manual Positioning

B. Airway Adjuncts

    1. Oropharyngeal airway

    2. Nasopharyngeal airway

C. Suction

IV. Artificial Ventilation

    A. Mouth-to-Mask With Supplemental Oxygen Technique

    B. Two-Person Bag-Valve-Mask Technique

    C. Flow-Restricted, Oxygen-Powered Ventilation Device

    D. One-Person Bag-Valve-Mask Technique

    E. Considerations for Trauma Patients

    F. Assessing the Adequacy of Artificial Ventilation

V. Special Situations in Airway Management

    A. Patients With Laryngectomies

    B. Ventilating Infants and Children

    C. Facial Injuries

    D. Obstructions

    E. Dental Appliances

● MATCHING

Match the terms in Column 1 with the correct definition in Column 2:

Column 1	Column 2
1. _____ Airway	a. the passageway into the trachea from the pharynx
2. _____ Alveoli	b. respiratory system structures through which air passes
3. _____ Bag-valve-mask (BVM)	c. the two major branches of the trachea into each lung
4. _____ Bronchi	d. causes the patient to retch when the throat is stimulated
5. _____ Cricoid ring	e. prevents food and liquid from entering the trachea
6. _____ Cyanotic	f. the air sacs in the lungs where gas exchange takes place
7. _____ Diaphragm	g. muscle separating the thoracic from the abdominal cavity
8. _____ Epiglottis	h. color of mucous membranes caused by hypoperfusion
9. _____ Gag reflex	i. muscles located between the ribs that move with breathing
10. _____ Glottis	j. a firm cartilage ring just inferior to lower portion of the larynx
11. _____ Intercostal muscles	k. voice box; consists of cartilage that vibrates when we speak
12. _____ Jaw thrust	l. surgical procedure in which the larynx is removed
13. _____ Laryngectomy	m. opening the airway by displacing the mandible forward
14. _____ Larynx	n. devices that remove secretions and fluids from the airway
15. _____ Nasal cannula	o. device for delivering oxygen from tubing into nostrils
16. _____ Nasopharyngeal airway	p. permanent artificial opening in the trachea
17. _____ Nasopharynx	q. inserted into mouth to lift the tongue out of the oropharynx
18. _____ Nonrebreather mask	r. high-flow device for delivering oxygen to the patient
19. _____ Oropharyngeal airway	s. ventilation device with a bag, a one-way valve, and a mask
20. _____ Oropharynx	t. the part of the airway behind the nose and mouth
21. _____ Pharynx	u. part of the pharynx behind the nose
22. _____ Suction devices	v. flexible tube inserted into the nostril to provide an air passage
23. _____ Trachea	w. the part of the airway behind the mouth
24. _____ Tracheal stoma	x. the windpipe

25. Label Figure 7-1 with the following terms:

nasopharynx   oropharynx
diaphragm   left bronchus
larynx   epiglottis
right bronchus

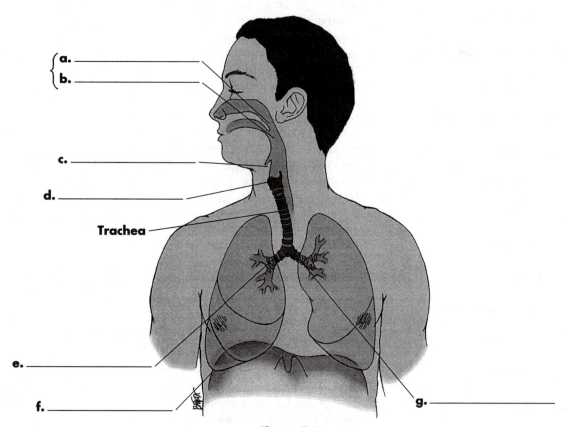

a.
b.
c.
d.
Trachea
e.
f.
g.

Figure 7-1

26. Label Figure 7-2 with the following terms:

one-way valve   oxygen reservoir valve
face mask   oxygen supply
self-inflating bag   oxygen reservoir

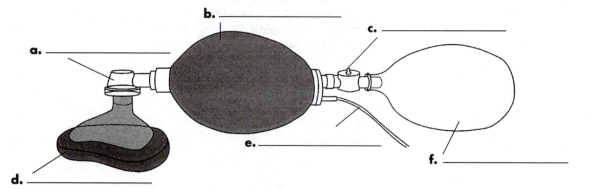

a.
b.
c.
d.
e.
f.

Figure 7-2

● REVIEW QUESTIONS

1. Inspiration flattens the diaphragm, pulling air into the lungs through the nose and mouth. **True or false?**
2. Exhalation and inhalation are considered active processes. **True or false?**
3. The normal range of respiratory rates for an adult is:
   a. 10-12   c. 12-20
   b. 12-30   d. 15-18
4. Indicate which of the following are signs and symptoms of inadequate breathing and which are signs of adequate breathing:

   _____ regular rhythm   _____ equal chest expansion

   _____ shortness of breath   _____ pale, cyanotic skin

   _____ decreased breath sounds   _____ slow rate

   _____ quiet breathing
5. What equipment is necessary to deliver oxygen to a patient?

   a. _____

   b. _____

   c. _____
6. What are the two types of oxygen delivery devices commonly used by EMT–Basics?

   a. _____

   b. _____
7. Nonrebreather masks can deliver up to _____ oxygen at 15 L/min.
   a. 97%   c. 90%
   b. 92%   d. 100%
8. Like the nonrebreather mask, the nasal cannula delivers high oxygen concentrations to the patient, and therefore is a good alternative to the nonrebreather mask. **True or false?**
9. The flow rate of a nasal cannula can be set to a maximum of _____ L/min.
   a. 2   c. 6
   b. 4   d. 8
10. The most common method of opening the airway for a trauma patient is the head-tilt, chin-lift technique. **True or false?**
11. List the steps in performing the head-tilt, chin-lift technique and the jaw thrust maneuver:

    Head-tilt, chin-lift- _____

    _____

    Jaw thrust- _____

    _____
12. Oral airways are measured from the corner of the mouth to the

    _____ or the _____.

13. How would you insert an oral airway for a child?
    a. Upside down, then gently rotate into place
    b. Right side up, using a tongue depressor
    c. Right side up, without a tongue depressor
    d. Oral airways are not recommended for children under 16 years of age
14. The nasal airway is preferred for patients who have a gag reflex. **True or false?**
15. The nasal airway is measured from the tip of the nose to the

    _____. The airway is inserted with the bevel toward

    the _____ of the nose.
16. If the EMT–Basic hears gurgling when assessing the patient's breathing, what should be done?

    _____

    _____

17. Which statement about the rigid suction catheter is **NOT** true?
    a. Easy to control
    b. Should be inserted until you can no longer see the tip
    c. Can be used on unresponsive patients
    d. Also called tonsil tip
18. Which of the following statements about bulb syringes is true?
    a. Used to suction the mouth and nose
    b. Inserted into the nostril and then compressed
    c. Dangerous to use for infants and children
    d. Can only be used for newborns up to 2 days of age
19. Suctioning should never last more than _____ before applying more oxygen.
    a. 15 seconds   c. 30 seconds
    b. 20 seconds   d. 1 minute
20. List the steps in performing mouth-to-mouth ventilation:

    _____

    _____

21. Mouth-to-mask is the preferred ventilation method because:
    a. Only one hand is used to form a mask seal
    b. It requires two people to ventilate the patient
    c. It provides excellent ventilatory volumes
    d. There is no need to use an oxygen source with the mask
22. Which of the following statements is true regarding one- and two-person bag-valve-mask techniques?
    a. With two people, one person maintains the mask seal and squeezes the bag and the second maintains an open airway
    b. With two people, one person maintains the mask seal and the second squeezes the bag
    c. The one-person technique is preferred when it is difficult to maintain the mask seal
    d. With the one- and two-person techniques, ventilate adult patients every second until the chest rises
23. The flow-restricted, oxygen-powered ventilation device:
    a. Can deliver oxygen at 65 L/min
    b. Does not require the EMT–Basic to maintain a mask seal
    c. Is safe for infants and children
    d. Delivers 100% oxygen when the trigger is pushed

38

24. Which of the following is a modification that must be made when ventilating a trauma patient?
    a. Use the head-tilt, chin-lift technique
    b. The EMT–Basic maintaining the mask seal also performs the jaw thrust
    c. Seal the mask over the bridge of nose and well below the chin
    d. The adult patient should be ventilated every 3 seconds
25. Indicate with an "A" which of the following statements describe signs of adequate ventilation when using a BVM. Indicate with an "I" which statements describe inadequate ventilation when using a BVM.

    _____ Chest rises and falls with each ventilation

    _____ The ventilatory rate is less than 12 times per minute

    _____ Skin color is cyanotic

    _____ Heart rate returns to normal

    _____ Chest does not rise with each ventilation

    _____ The stomach becomes distended
26. Place in order the following steps in correcting poor chest rise during ventilation, with 1 as the first step and 4 as the last:

    _____ Check mask seal   _____ Reposition the jaw

    _____ Try different technique   _____ Check for an obstruction
27. How would you ventilate a patient who has a tracheal stoma?

    _____

    _____

28. Oral airways should never be used on trauma patients. **True or false?**
29. If at all possible, try to leave dentures and other dental appliances in place. They add shape and structure, making it easier to create a mask seal. **True or false?**
30. You have been dispatched to the home of a sick child. On arrival, the child's mother tells you that her 3-year-old daughter awoke from sleep with a barking cough. The patient is sitting in her father's lap and is leaning forward to breathe.
    a. What are important anatomic and physiologic considerations to keep in mind when caring for a pediatric patient with difficulty breathing?

    _____

    _____

    _____

    b. What are the signs and symptoms of inadequate breathing?

    _____

    _____

    _____

c. What is tidal volume and what is the easiest way to evaluate it?

_____

_____

_____

31. You and your partner are using a two-person bag-valve-mask technique to ventilate an unresponsive patient. During your assessment, you notice that the patient's skin color is not improving. You reposition the patient's jaw and check the mask seal, yet the patient's chest rise remains inadequate.
   a. What are the signs and symptoms of adequate ventilation that should be monitored while providing artificial ventilation?

_____

_____

   b. You decide to try an alternative method to ventilate this patient. What method would you choose?

_____

_____

   c. Alternative methods do not correct the patient's inadequate chest rise. What should you do next?

_____

_____

Directions: Circle the letter of the correct answer.

1. Which of the following occurs during inhalation?
   a. The diaphragm relaxes
   c. The chest expands
   b. The diaphragm raises
   d. The ribs move downward and inward

2. Which of the following is the average breathing rate in children?
   a. 12-20 breaths per minute
   c. 25-50 breaths per minute
   b. 15-30 breaths per minute
   d. 12-50 breaths per minute

3. Which of the following is characteristic of adequate breathing?
   a. Irregular rhythm
   b. Diminished or absent breath sounds
   c. Shallow respirations
   d. Equal chest expansion

4. A patient presents with difficulty breathing, a respiratory rate of 20 breaths per minute, and cyanotic mucous membranes. The patient says that he is on oxygen at home via nasal cannula at 4 L/min. How would you deliver oxygen to the patient?
   a. Nasal cannula at 2-4 L/min
   b. Nasal cannula at 6 L/min
   c. Nonrebreather mask at 6 L/min
   d. Nonrebreather mask at 12-15 L/min

5. How should the airway be opened on a patient with suspected cervical spine injury?
   a. Head-tilt
   c. Jaw thrust
   b. Head-tilt, chin lift
   d. Hyperextension of head

6. Which of the following is appropriate when measuring or inserting an oral airway?
   a. Use oral airways in unresponsive patients with a gag reflex
   b. Oral airways are measured for size from the tip of the nose to corner of the jaw
   c. Oral airways are inserted upside down until the flange reaches the teeth, then rotated
   d. Oral airways may be inserted by using a tongue depressor

7. How far should the suction catheter tip be inserted into the patient's mouth?
   a. Just to the front teeth
   c. To the molars
   b. To the central incisors
   d. Only as far as you can see

8. What should be done if large amounts of emesis or secretions are present in the patient's airway?
   a. Log roll the patient and clear the airway
   b. Suction for up to 1 minute, then ventilate
   c. Place the patient in the prone position
   d. Ventilate the patient first, then suction

9. What is the maximum length of time to suction a patient between ventilations?
   a. 5 seconds
   c. 15 seconds
   b. 10 seconds
   d. 20 seconds

10. Place the four methods of ventilation in order of preference, with 1 as the most preferred method and 4 as the least.

_____ One-person, bag-valve-mask

_____ Mouth-to-mask

_____ Flow-restricted, oxygen-powered ventilation device

_____ Two-person, bag-valve-mask

11. Which of the following is **NOT** true of the bag-valve-mask?
    a. Has a self-inflating bag
    b. Has a pop-off valve set at 40 L/min
    c. Has standardized 15/22-mm adapter
    d. Is available in infant, child, and adult sizes

12. Which of the following statements is true concerning a flow-restricted, oxygen-powered ventilation device?
    a. A peak flow rate of 80% oxygen occurs at 60 L/min
    b. Relief valve opens at approximately 100 cm of water
    c. An alarm sounds when relief valve pressure is exceeded
    d. The EMT–Basic can use only one hand to ventilate the patient

13. When using a bag-valve-mask on a trauma patient with suspected spinal injury, which of the following is an accepted technique of ventilation?
    a. Stabilize the head and neck before ventilation
    b. Use the ring finger and little finger to bring jaw forward to the mask while tilting the head
    c. A head-tilt, chin-lift should be performed to allow for best ventilation
    d. Ventilate every 3 seconds for adults, children, and infants

14. Which of the following is a special consideration when ventilating infants and children?
    a. The head needs to be tilted further back for children and infants
    b. Avoid excessive pressure when using the BVM
    c. Gastric distention is less common in children
    d. Use a BVM with a pop-off valve

15. What should you do if dentures become dislodged while you are ventilating a patient?
    a. Leave them in place
    b. Take them out
    c. Pull up on the jaw to hold them in place
    d. Take out the upper teeth

DIVISION THREE
PATIENT ASSESSMENT

CHAPTER 8

SCENE SIZE-UP

● **CHAPTER OUTLINE**

   I. Body Substance Isolation Precautions

   II. Scene Safety

      A. Personal Protection

      B. Protection of the Patient

      C. Protection of Bystanders

   III. Nature of Illness and Mechanism of Injury

      A. Nature of Illness

      B. Trauma Patients

   IV. Number of Patients and Need for Additional Help

● MATCHING

Match the terms in Column 1 with the correct definition in Column 2:

	Column 1		Column 2
1.	_____ Mechanism of injury	a.	patient's description of the chief complaint, or why EMS was called
2.	_____ Nature of illness	b.	evaluation of the entire environment for possible risks to yourself, crew members, patients, or bystanders
3.	_____ Scene size-up	c.	event or forces that caused the damage to the patient

● REVIEW QUESTIONS

1. Personal protection includes body substance isolation precautions and appropriate clothing for the environment and situation. **True or false?**
2. Scene safety includes all of the following **EXCEPT:**
   a. Bystander protection
   b. Evaluation prior to entering the scene
   c. Patient assessment
   d. Evaluation of the entire scene for danger
3. List three hazards that may be present at the scene of an automobile crash:

   a. _____

   b. _____

   c. _____
4. What types of hazards may be present at the scene of a medical call?

   _____

   _____
5. How would you determine if the scene was safe to enter?

   _____

   _____
6. The most important statement to remember concerning scene safety is:

   _____

   _____
7. The nature of illness is also called the _____.
   a. Chief complaint   c. Mechanism of injury
   b. Past medical history   d. Patient assessment
8. You can usually determine the mechanism of injury for a trauma patient by looking at the surroundings. **True or false?**
9. Why is it important to identify the mechanism of injury for a trauma patient?

   _____

   _____

10. Why is it important to determine the total number of patients at the scene?

_____

_____

11. List three reasons to request additional help:

a. _____

b. _____

c. _____

12. You have been dispatched to a domestic quarrel where "shots have been fired." En route, you are advised by dispatch that police have secured the scene and that it is safe to enter.

a. Based on this information, what preparations should you make while responding to the scene?

_____

_____

b. On arrival in the area, you are escorted to the scene by law enforcement personnel. What are your priorities in managing this scene?

_____

_____

c. While assessing a woman who has been shot in the abdomen, the perpetrator breaks away from police custody. What should you do?

_____

_____

13. You have responded to a motor vehicle crash involving three cars and multiple patients. Fire and rescue personnel are en route, but your crew is first to arrive at the scene.

a. What are your responsibilities during the scene size-up?

_____

_____

b. Using your senses of vision, smell, and sound, how would you evaluate this scene for safety?

_____

_____

c. What are your responsibilities in protecting a patient from further injury during extrication?

_____

_____

INITIAL ASSESSMENT

● **CHAPTER OUTLINE**

● REVIEW QUESTIONS

1. List two reasons for forming a general impression of the patient:

   a. _____

   b. _____

2. The general impression should include all of the following **EXCEPT**:
   - **a.** Age, gender, race
   - **b.** Name
   - **c.** Mechanism of injury
   - **d.** Nature of illness

3. Because young children cannot answer questions, there is usually no way to determine the level of their mental status. **True or false?**

4. How would you assess if a patient was alert, responsive to verbal stimuli, responsive to painful stimuli, or unresponsive?

   _____

   _____

5. Changes in mental status are a late indication of a change in patient condition. **True or false?**

6. The head-tilt, chin-lift is used for _____ patients, and the jaw thrust is used for _____ patients.
   - **a.** Medical; unresponsive
   - **b.** Trauma; medical
   - **c.** Medical; trauma
   - **d.** Unresponsive; uncooperative

7. Why is the head manually stabilized in the neutral position for trauma patients?

   _____

8. EMT–Basics should administer oxygen to an adult patient breathing less

   than _____ times per minute or greater

   than _____ times per minute. If the patient is breathing adequately but is unresponsive, help maintain a(n)

   _____ airway and administer _____ oxygen.

9. How would you determine if a patient was breathing and evaluate breathing efforts?

   _____

10. When assessing the breathing of an infant, assessing the rate is of little importance compared with assessing the quality, and no care needs to be provided for changes in rate. **True or false?**

11. Immediately after completing the initial assessment, EMT–Basics should care for any life-threatening injuries found. **True or false?**

12. Initially assess the adult patient's pulse by palpating the _____ artery, the child's pulse by palpating the _____ artery, and an infant's pulse by palpating the _____ artery.
    - **a.** Radial; radial; brachial
    - **b.** Radial; brachial; brachial
    - **c.** Carotid; carotid; radial
    - **d.** Carotid; brachial; radial

13. The first time the EMT–Basic assesses for external bleeding is during the

_____ _____ and assesses for external

bleeding again when evaluating the patient's _____.

14. List three abnormal skin colors, three abnormal skin temperatures, and three abnormal skin conditions:

Color _____

Temperature _____

Condition _____

15. Capillary refill should be less than 3 seconds when evaluating infants and children. **True or false?**

16. Which of the following situations constitutes a priority patient?
   a. Uncomplicated childbirth
   b. Severe abdominal pain
   c. Unresponsive patient with an intact gag reflex
   d. Chest pain and blood pressure less than 150 systolic

17. Why do EMT–Basics determine if a patient has a priority condition during the initial assessment?

18. You have been dispatched to a motorcycle crash. Police are on the scene, and the scene is safe. On arrival, you find a teenage boy lying in the road.
   a. What are seven elements of patient evaluation to consider during the initial assessment?

_____

_____

_____

   b. The patient is lying on his left side. There are blood, vomit, and broken teeth in his mouth. How will you manage his airway?

_____

_____

_____

   c. The patient is not responsive to verbal stimulus but withdraws appropriately from painful stimulus. How would you describe this patient's level of responsiveness?

_____

_____

_____

19. Your EMS crew is caring for three patients who were victims of a drive-by shooting. The first patient is a 15-year-old girl who was grazed on the upper arm by a passing bullet. She is hysterical and is difficult to assess. The second patient is a 27-year-old man who was shot in the chest and has lost a large amount of blood. The third patient is a 54-year-old woman who has a wound to her lower back and is unable to feel or move her lower extremities.

a. Based on your initial assessment, which of these patients is a "priority patient" who should be rapidly transported?

_____

_____

b. Because your ambulance is the only one on the scene, how would you arrange for rapid transport of the priority patient?

_____

_____

c. Define ways to identify priority patients.

_____

_____

CHAPTER 10

FOCUSED HISTORY AND PHYSICAL EXAMINATION FOR TRAUMA PATIENTS

● **CHAPTER OUTLINE**

I. Mechanism of Injury

II. Evaluating Patients With Serious Injuries or Mechanisms of Injury

    A. Performing the Rapid Trauma Assessment

    B. Baseline Vital Signs and SAMPLE History

III. Evaluating Patients With No Significant Mechanism of Injury

● MATCHING

Match the terms in Column 1 with the correct definition in Column 2:

Column 1	Column 2
1. _____ Crepitation	a. system in which care is provided at basic and advanced levels
2. _____ DCAP-BTLS	b. testing the ability to move
3. _____ Distal pulse	c. grating or crackling sound or sensation
4. _____ Iliac wings	d. ability to feel a touch against the skin
5. _____ Jugular vein distention	e. pulse taken away from the center of the body (*ie*, wrist)
6. _____ Motor function	f. anteriosuperior tips of the pelvis
7. _____ Multitiered response system	g. acronym standing for the eight components of assessment
8. _____ Paradoxical Motion	h. abnormal enlargement of the blood vessels on the sides of the neck
9. _____ Sensation	i. abnormal movement of the chest wall during inspiration and exhalation in which the affected portion moves opposite the unaffected portion

● REVIEW QUESTIONS

1. Explain why it is important to identify the mechanism of injury:

_____

_____

2. Which of the following is **NOT** considered a high-risk mechanism of injury?
   a. Ejection
   b. Fall from a 6-foot ladder
   c. Motorcycle crash
   d. Vehicle/pedestrian collision
3. Elderly patients, infants, and children can be more easily injured than healthy adults. **True or false?**
4. Fill in the blanks with the appropriate term from the DCAP-BTLS acronym:

D _____   B _____

C _____   T _____

A _____   L _____

P _____   S _____

5. The rapid trauma assessment should take approximately _____ seconds.
6. What should you do if you discover any life-threatening conditions during the rapid trauma assessment?

_____

_____

7. Breath sounds are auscultated at the _____ at the midclavicular line and _____ at the midaxillary line.
   a. Clavicles; ribs
   c. Upper quadrant; lower quadrant
   b. Apices; bases
   d. Lungs; intercostal space
8. At rest, most patients will have a _____ abdomen.
   a. Soft
   c. Rigid
   b. Firm
   d. Tender
9. Which of the following best describes the motions used in evaluation of the pelvis?
   a. Rock and tilt
   c. Flex and compress
   b. Squeeze and tilt
   d. Flex and squeeze
10. The extremities must be evaluated for DCAP-BTLS as well as _____. (Mark all that are appropriate)

   _____ Sensation   _____ Motor function

   _____ Distal pulses   _____ Flexion

   _____ Response to deep pain   _____ Extension
11. For patients who have sustained a serious mechanism of injury but who complain only of an isolated injury, the assessment should be focused on the isolated injury. **True or false?**
12. Every trauma patient should receive a rapid trauma assessment. **True or false?**
13. Patients generally know when they have a more serious underlying injury that is not apparent. **True or false?**

For questions 14 through 16, indicate which patients should receive a rapid trauma assessment (R) and which should receive a focused history and physical examination directed only toward the injury (F).

14. _____ 10-year-old girl who was hit by her brother in the forearm with a rake

15. _____ 47-year-old woman who twisted her ankle when stepping off the curb

16. _____ 28-year-old man who fell off a roof while working and is up walking around at the scene and states he is not injured

17. You and your crew have been dispatched to a construction site where a worker has fallen from the roof of a two-story building. On arrival, you find a 30-year-old man lying supine on the ground. He is responsive and alert and tells you that "he is fine." His supervisor is trying to persuade him to go to the hospital.
   a. Would this patient be considered at high risk for hidden injury? Why or why not?

   _____

   b. What questions would you ask this patient as you obtain a focused history?

   _____

   c. Following your initial assessment, how would you prepare this patient for transport?

   _____

18. Your crew is one of three EMS units that has been dispatched to an explosion at a chemical plant. En route, you are advised that there are five patients with serious injuries. Police and fire and rescue personnel have secured the scene and made it safe. The patient for whom you are caring is an unresponsive 47-year-old woman. She has obvious soft-tissue injuries and is breathing with gurgling respirations.

a. What is your first priority in managing this patient?

_____

_____

b. Because you suspect a head injury, what steps would you take before initiating the rapid trauma assessment?

_____

_____

c. Describe the head-to-toe assessment you would perform on this patient and how you would evaluate her for injury using DCAP-BTLS.

_____

_____

CHAPTER 11

FOCUSED HISTORY AND PHYSICAL EXAMINATION FOR MEDICAL PATIENTS

● **CHAPTER OUTLINE**

I. Responsive Medical Patients

    A. The Patient's History

    B. Rapid Assessment

    C. Vital Signs

    D. Emergency Care

II. Unresponsive Medical Patients

● MATCHING

Match the terms in Column 1 with the correct definition in Column 2:

	Column 1		Column 2
1. _____	OPQRST	a.	acronym for eliciting patient information about a particular condition
2. _____	Provocation	b.	quick evaluation of the patient, accomplished in 60 to 90 seconds
3. _____	Rapid assessment	c.	term referring to something that induces a physical reaction
4. _____	SAMPLE history	d.	acronym used to evaluate a patient's past medical condition and current events

● REVIEW QUESTIONS

1. Responsive and unresponsive medical patients receive the same focused history and physical examination. **True or false?**

2. Fill in the blanks with the correct terms of the OPQRST acronym:

   O _____

   P _____

   Q _____

   R _____

   S _____

   T _____

Using the appropriate letter of the OPQRST acronym, indicate which component of the patient information is represented for questions 3 through 9:

3. _____ What position makes you feel better?

4. _____ How long have you had cardiac problems?

5. _____ How long have you had this pain?

6. _____ Is this the worst pain you have ever had?

7. _____ What makes the pain worse?

8. _____ Does the pain spread or move?

9. _____ Can you describe the pain you are feeling?

10. A SAMPLE history should be done on every patient. **True or false?**

11. Fill in the blanks with the correct terms of the SAMPLE acronym:

S _____

A _____

M _____

P _____

L _____

E _____

12. The focused history and physical examination for the medical patient is

guided by the patient's _____ _____.

13. Why is it important to find out if the patient has a known medical problem during the focused history and physical examination of the medical patient? How might the history of a medical problem change the EMT–Basic's care for this patient?

_____

_____

14. Unresponsive medical patients should be evaluated using the rapid trauma assessment. **True or false?**

15. When a medical patient is unresponsive and cannot provide a SAMPLE

history, information can be obtained from _____.

16. Which of the following positions is appropriate for the unresponsive medical patient without spinal trauma?
   a. Fowler's   **c.** Recovery
   b. Trendelenburg   **d.** Supine

17. You are caring for a 58-year-old man complaining of chest pain. He is alert and oriented and tells you that he thinks he is having a "heart attack." As your partner applies high-concentration oxygen and obtains vital signs, you begin to gather a patient history using the OPQRST acronym.
   a. What does the "O" signify, and what questions would be appropriate to ask this patient?

_____

_____

_____

   b. What does the "Q" signify, and what questions would be appropriate to ask this patient?

_____

_____

_____

c. What does the "T" signify, and what questions would be appropriate to ask this patient?

_____

_____

_____

18. You have been dispatched to a local shopping mall for an "unresponsive woman." On arrival, you find a young woman lying on the floor in a department store. Bystanders state that the woman "just collapsed." No other patient information is available.

a. What are your first priorities in managing this patient?

_____

_____

_____

b. How would you assess this patient?

_____

_____

_____

c. If you could be certain there was no trauma present, how would you transport this patient?

_____

_____

_____

CHAPTER 12

DETAILED PHYSICAL EXAMINATION

● **CHAPTER OUTLINE**

● REVIEW QUESTIONS

1. The purpose of the detailed physical examination is to gather details that may have been missed on the rapid trauma assessment. **True or False?**

2. The detailed physical examination is a routine part of the assessment for all trauma patients. **True or False?**

3. A patient involved in a rollover vehicle crash complains only of pain in her left lower leg and foot. This patient would still require a detailed physical examination. **True or False?**

4. When would a detailed physical examination be indicated for a medical patient?

_____

_____

5. Fill in the blanks with then appropriate terms of the DCAP-BTLS acronym:

D _____		B _____
C _____		T _____
A _____		L _____
P _____		S _____

6. The ambient light in the ambulance is adequate for evaluating the ears and nose for drainage and inspecting the mouth. **True or False?**

7. When evaluating the neck, you should assess for DCAP-BTLS and

_____ .

8. What conditions might lead an EMT–Basic to choose not flex and compress a patient's pelvis?

_____

_____

9. The best time to perform the detailed physical examination is:
   a. On scene, prior to transport
   b. In the back of the ambulance, prior to transport
   c. In the back of the ambulance, during transport
   d. At the receiving facility

10. You are caring for an 8-year-old girl who has fallen from a treehouse. The child fell approximately 10 feet and landed on the grassy surface below the tree. She is alert and crying, and there are no apparent injuries.
    a. After completing the focused history and physical examination for a trauma patient, would this require a detailed physical examination?

_____

_____

    b. What are the eight components of the examination procedure that should be evaluated?

_____

_____

c. Based on the mechanism of injury, during the focused history and physical exaination, how would you evaluate the patient's neck?

_____

_____

11. You have been dispatched to a local restaurant where a waiter has been burned by hot coffee. Your initial assessment reveals superficial and partial thickness burns to the patient's right hand and forearm. He is responsive, alert, and in extreme pain.

a. Should this patient receive a detailed physical examination?

_____

_____

b. How would you evaluate this patient's injury?

_____

_____

c. Would you assess vital signs on this patient?

_____

_____

CHAPTER 13

ONGOING ASSESSMENT

● **CHAPTER OUTLINE**

I. Components of the Ongoing Assessment

II. Repeat the Initial Assessment

III. Repeat Vital Signs and Focused Assessment

IV. Check Interventions

● REVIEW QUESTIONS

1. List three purposes of the ongoing assessment:

   a. _____

   b. _____

   c. _____

2. What are the components of the initial assessment that are repeated during the ongoing assessment?

   _____

   _____

3. How frequently do you reassess a stable patient? _____

4. Number the following steps in the ongoing assessment, with 1 as the first step and 6 as the last:

   _____ Assess skin color, temperature, condition, perfusion

   _____ Assess mental status

   _____ Assess pulse

   _____ Assess airway patency

   _____ Assess breathing rate and quality

   _____ Reassess patient priority

5. The focused assessment of the chief complaint is not part of the ongoing assessment. **True or false?**

6. Why is it important to document successive sets of vital signs over time? What is this process called?

   _____

   _____

7. List three examples of interventions that the EMT–Basic should evaluate during the ongoing assessment:

   a. _____

   b. _____

   c. _____

8. You are en route to the emergency department with a trauma patient who was a victim of a "hit-and-run" automobile-pedestrian collision. The patient is responsive to verbal stimulus, has multiple injuries, and is fully immobilized on a long spine board.

   a. How often should the ongoing assessment of this patient be performed?

   _____

   _____

b. As part of your ongoing assessment, how will you reassess the patient's mental status?

_____

_____

c. If the patient becomes unresponsive, how will you continue to assess his mental status?

_____

_____

9. You are caring for a 78-year-old woman with difficulty breathing. She has a history of "heart failure" and is in moderate respiratory distress. You have applied high-concentration oxygen via a nonrebreather mask and allowed her to assume a position of comfort. Her vital signs are: blood pressure 146/88, pulse 134 strong and regular, respirations 28 labored and noisy. En route to the emergency department you check your interventions.

a. How will you ensure the concentration of oxygen delivery?

_____

_____

b. How can you check your method of oxygen delivery?

_____

_____

c. What should you do if the patient cannot tolerate the face mask?

_____

_____

CHAPTER 14

COMMUNICATIONS

● **CHAPTER OUTLINE**

I. Communication Systems and Components

    A. Communication Components

    B. System Maintenance

II. Procedures for Radio Communications

    A. Communication With Dispatch

    B. Communication With Medical Direction

    C. Verbal Communication

III. Interpersonal Communication

    A. General Principles

    B. Tips for Effective Communication

    C. Special Populations

● MATCHING

Match the terms in Column 1 with the correct definition in Column 2:

Column 1	Column 2
1. _____ Base station	**a.** transmission or exchange of information, ideas, and skills through language, body movements, etc.
2. _____ Communication	**b.** digital radio equipment that allows the user to block out radio transmissions that are not intended for that unit
3. _____ Encoders and decoders	**c.** radio transceiver located at a stationary site, such as a hospital, mountain top, or dispatch center
4. _____ Repeater	**d.** remote receiver that receives a transmission from a low-power portable or mobile radio on one frequency and then transmits the signal at a higher power, often on another frequency

● REVIEW QUESTIONS

1. A radio at a stationary site with superior transmission and receiving capabilities is called a:
   - **a.** Repeater
   - **b.** Base station
   - **c.** Transceiver
   - **d.** Encoder

2. The agency that regulates and monitors radio transmissions is called the

   _____.

3. You should monitor the radio frequency for _____ seconds before transmitting to ensure that the frequency is clear.

4. How long should you wait to begin speaking after pushing the push-to-talk button?
   - **a.** 1 second
   - **b.** 3 seconds
   - **c.** 5 seconds
   - **d.** 10 seconds

5. The phrase _____ means to wait before continuing with the transmission.

6. Use everyday language during radio communication to reduce confusion. **True or false?**

7. Courtesy is an important part of radio communications, so be sure to use "please" and "thank you" on a regular basis. **True or false?**

8. Which of the following is **NOT** a routine part of communications with dispatch?
   - **a.** Receiving the call
   - **b.** Arriving at the receiving facility
   - **c.** Loading the patient at the scene
   - **d.** Arriving at the scene

9. An effective radio report should be _____.
   - **a.** Comprehensive
   - **b.** Concise
   - **c.** Patterned
   - **d.** Lengthy

10. List the 12 components included in the standard medical reporting format in order:

a. _____

b. _____

c. _____

d. _____

e. _____

f. _____

g. _____

h. _____

i. _____

j. _____

k. _____

l. _____

11. List three tips for effective communication:

a. _____

b. _____

c. _____

12. Body language consists of things such as posture, facial expressions, and tone of voice. **True or false?**

13. You have been dispatched to a local bowling alley for a "possible heart attack." On arrival, you find an unresponsive woman in her mid-forties lying on the floor of the bathroom. She is breathing and has a pulse of 124. Her blood pressure is 108/64. No other information is available. As your partner monitors her airway, you contact medical direction via a cellular phone.

a. What information should you include about this patient in your initial report to the hospital?

_____

_____

b. At the end of your radio report, what should you do before you end your transmission?

_____

_____

c. The medical direction physician recommended an intervention that was unclear to you and your partner. What should you do?

_____

_____

14. You have responded to a crash scene involving a school bus and a city transportation vehicle for the elderly. The students on the bus are from a private school for the physically challenged. There appears to be no major injuries, but the students and elderly passengers are frightened and some are hysterical.

a. What are some general considerations to keep in mind when dealing with ill or injured children?

_____

_____

b. What are some general considerations to keep in mind when dealing with elderly patients?

_____

_____

c. Several of the children are hearing impaired. What are ways to communicate with these patients?

_____

_____

CHAPTER 15

DOCUMENTATION

● **CHAPTER OUTLINE**

   I. Minimum Data Set

  II. The Prehospital Care Report

      A. Functions of the Prehospital Care Report

      B. Traditional Format

      C. Other Formats

      D. Distribution

      E. Documentation of Patient Care Errors

      F. Correction of Documentation Errors

 III. Documentation of Patient Refusal

 IV. Special Situations

      A. Multiple Casualty Incidents

      B. Special Situation Reports

● MATCHING

Match the terms in Column 1 with the correct definition in Column 2:

	Column 1		Column 2
1. _____	Administrative information	a.	essential elements of patient and administrative data required for accurate and complete prehospital data collection
2. _____	Minimum data set		
3. _____	Patient information	b.	section of a prehospital care report that allows EMT–Basics to document information using a standard medical reporting format
4. _____	Patient narrative		
5. _____	Prehospital care report	c.	process of comparing serial recordings of a patient's vital signs or other assessments to note changes
6. _____	Trending		
		d.	elements such as time of dispatch and location of call related to the prehospital care call
		e.	elements such as patient's clinical condition and chief complaint related to the prehospital care call
		f.	form used to document the events occurring during a patient encounter

● REVIEW QUESTIONS

1. Trending information requires that the same sets of information be collected and recorded over a period of time. **True or false?**
2. All of the following are elements of the patient information data set **EXCEPT:**
   a. Injury description
   b. Skin color, temperature, and condition
   c. Chief complaint
   d. Time of arrival at patient
3. Write the following times in a 24-hour format:

   1 AM _____   6:30 PM _____

   12 noon _____   4:20 AM _____

   10:30 PM _____   8:25 PM _____

   2:40 AM _____   12:30 AM _____

4. The prehospital care report is both a legal and medical document. **True or false?**
5. Place an 'S' next to statements that are subjective and an 'O' next to statements that are objective.

   _____ I saw him drinking at that bar

   _____ The patient was drunk

   _____ It looked like the car was going over the speed limit

   _____ Her blood pressure was 120/80 and the pulse was 72

   _____ The patient's skin is cool, clammy, and moist to the touch

6. Name three things, other than documenting patient care, for which the pre-hospital care report can be used:

   a. _____

   b. _____

   c. _____

7. Most prehospital care report forms have a section for writing a patient

   _____, allowing EMT–Basics to write about the events in the standard medical reporting format.

8. Write the common abbreviations for these terms:

   Chief complaint _____   Gunshot wound _____

   Every _____   Shortness of breath _____

   History _____   Immediately _____

   Treatment _____   Alcohol _____

9. Correct errors in documentation by scratching out the wrong information and filling in the correct information. **True or false?**

10. Refusal is the right of any _____ adult, meaning any adult who can make rational decisions about his/her care.

11. List at least three reasons to use a special situation report:

    a. _____

    b. _____

    c. _____

12. You have been asked to assist a neighboring EMS agency in developing a minimum data set of information to be collected by their employees during emergency and nonemergency responses.

    a. What are the two categories of information contained in a minimum data set

    _____

    _____

    b. What components should be included when gathering patient care information?

    _____

    _____

    _____

c. What components should be included when gathering information for administrative purposes?

_____

_____

_____

13. You have been dispatched to a local diner for a "possible allergic reaction." On arrival, you find a man in his mid-thirties. He is alert and aggravated with the manager for calling EMS. The patient tells you he was feeling a little weak and nauseated and had some trouble catching his breath. He is sure that it is just "a touch of the flu." He refuses to be examined or transported to the hospital.

a. Does this patient have a legal right to refuse treatment?

_____

_____

_____

b. What might you do to persuade the patient to receive treatment and transportation to the hospital?

_____

_____

_____

c. The patient still refuses care. How should you complete this call?

_____

_____

_____

DIVISION THREE EXAMINATION
PATIENT ASSESSMENT

Directions: Circle the letter of the correct answer.

1. Which of the following statements is true regarding body substance isolation (BSI) precautions?
   a. BSI precautions protect the EMT–Basic from blood-borne pathogens only
   b. BSI precautions protect the EMT–Basic from air- and blood-borne pathogens
   c. The need for BSI precautions is determined during the initial assessment
   d. BSI precautions are necessary only when blood is present

2. Which of the following is the EMT–Basic's primary concern?
   a. Patient safety   c. Bystander safety
   b. Personal safety   d. Crew member safety

3. Which of the following information is obtained during the scene size-up?
   a. Mechanism of injury or nature of illness
   b. The patient's mental status
   c. Patient assessment
   d. The patient's airway, breathing, and circulatory status

4. During the scene size-up, the EMT–Basic should:
   a. Determine the number of patients at the scene
   b. Wait for additional help to arrive if there are too many patients to treat
   c. Begin to treat patients based on their mechanism of injury
   d. Determine scene safety after beginning patient care

5. The first phase of the initial assessment is the general impression. Which of the following is identified in the general impression?
   a. Assess mental status
   b. Assess respiratory effort
   c. Determine if any life threats are present
   d. Determine if pulse is present

6. What does the "P" in the acronym AVPU represent?
   a. Provocation   c. Partially responsive
   b. Responds to Painful stimuli   d. Priority patient

7. While assessing an unresponsive patient, the EMT–Basic determines the patient's respiratory rate is 6 per minute. What should be done at this time?
   a. Continue assessment from head to toe, then apply oxygen
   b. Continue the assessment to the abdomen, then give oxygen via a nonrebreather mask
   c. Have your partner ventilate the patient
   d. Immediately place the patient on oxygen at 12 to 15 L/min via a nonrebreather mask

8. Where would you initially assess the pulse for an alert adult patient?
   a. Carotid pulse   c. Femoral pulse
   b. Radial pulse   d. Brachial pulse

9. Where should the EMT–Basic evaluate the color of the patient's skin to assess perfusion?
   a. Nail beds   c. Scalp
   b. Abdomen   d. Extremities

10. Which of the following is an accurate assessment of the patient's perfusion?
    a. The color of the skin of the extremities
    b. The capillary refill of a 14-year-old boy
    c. The skin temperature of the patient's hand
    d. The comparison of the strength of the carotid and radial pulses in an adult

11. Which of the following is a priority patient requiring immediate care and transport?
    a. An unresponsive patient with no gag reflex
    b. A patient with chest pain and blood pressure of 138/84
    c. A responsive patient who can follow commands
    d. A patient who feels no pain in his obviously deformed ankle
12. Which of the following is considered a significant mechanism of injury?
    a. Death of another passenger in the same compartment
    b. Falls greater than 5 feet
    c. A vehicle crash at 15 miles per hour
    d. Penetrating injuries to the upper extremities
13. How long should it take to perform a rapid trauma assessment on most patients?
    a. 10 seconds   c. 60-90 seconds
    b. 10-30 seconds   d. 2-3 minutes
14. Which of the following is part of the acronym DCAP-BTLS?
    a. D = Deformity   c. T = Time
    b. A = Amputation   d. S = Severity of injury
15. During the rapid trauma assessment, assess the abdomen for DCAP-BTLS and:
    a. Paradoxical motion   c. Distention
    b. Crepitation   d. Instability
16. For a patient with a twisted ankle and no other injuries or mechanism to suggest injury, how would you assess the patient during the focused history and physical examination?
    a. Perform the rapid trauma assessment
    b. Assess the pelvis and both extremities
    c. Assess only the specific injury
    d. Perform the rapid trauma assessment after inspecting the injury
17. The acronym OPQRST helps EMT–Basics remember what questions to ask concerning:
    a. The patient's mechanism of injury
    b. The patient's mental status
    c. The patient's chief complaint
    d. The patient's history
18. Which of the following statements is true concerning the focused history and physical examination for the medical patient?
    a. Emergency care is based on signs and symptoms found, in consultation with medical direction
    b. Unresponsive medical patients are evaluated much the same as responsive medical patients
    c. Unresponsive medical patients with no signs of trauma should be placed in the prone position
    d. EMT–Basics do not need to perform an initial assessment on medical patients, so include an assessment of the airway, breathing, and circulation in the focused history and physical examination
19. In the SAMPLE acronym, S stands for:
    a. Signs and symptoms   c. Side effects
    b. Sensation   d. Severity of the illness
20. The rapid assessment for a responsive medical patient:
    a. Must include a head-to-toe assessment
    b. Requires removal of all patient clothing
    c. Is directed toward the patient's chief complaint
    d. Rules out the possibility of trauma

21. Which of the following is correct care for an unresponsive medical patient?
    a. Perform a trauma assessment only when there is known trauma
    b. Do not immobilize unless you are sure the patient's spine was injured
    c. Place the patient in the recovery position if you know the spine is injured
    d. Perform a rapid trauma assessment to determine illness or injury

22. Which of the following statements is true concerning the detailed physical examination?
    a. The detailed physical examination is performed more rapidly than the focused history and physical examination
    b. The detailed physical examination is designed for trauma patients who may have hidden injuries
    c. Ideally, the detailed physical examination should be performed on scene
    d. The detailed physical examination is most often performed on medical patients

23. Which patient would most likely receive a detailed physical examination?
    a. A responsive medical patient with no injuries
    b. A patient with an isolated injury and no serious mechanism of injury
    c. An unresponsive medical patient
    d. A medical patient with shortness of breath

24. When inspecting the head during the detailed physical examination, you will evaluate for the first time:
    a. The ears for drainage
    b. The pupil size and reactivity
    c. The airway
    d. The face for instability

25. Which of the following is true?
    a. Listen for breath sounds in two places, once at the apices on each side
    b. Assess the abdomen in two quadrants
    c. Assess the pelvis if there is sign of injury
    d. Assess the neck for jugular vein distention

26. When evaluating the extremities during the detailed physical examination, assess for DCAP-BTLS and distal:
    a. Pain
    b. Sensation
    c. Distention
    d. Crepitation

27. Which of the following is true concerning the ongoing assessment?
    a. Vital signs are assessed every 30 minutes during the ongoing assessment
    b. The ongoing assessment repeats the initial assessment except for the mental status check
    c. The ongoing assessment should be performed once during transport
    d. The ongoing assessment allows for evaluation of trends in the patient's condition

28. How often should ongoing assessments be performed on stable patients?
    a. Every 5 minutes
    b. Every 10 minutes
    c. Every 15 minutes
    d. Every 20 minutes

29. Which of the following is true?
    a. Any intervention that is inadequate should be removed
    b. The ongoing assessment should be repeated one last time about 5 minutes away from the receiving facility
    c. EMT–Basics should check interventions like pupil size and mental status
    d. The focused assessment does not have to be repeated as part of the ongoing assessment if the patient is unresponsive

30. Which organization regulates radio frequencies?
    a. FAA
    b. FCA
    c. FCC
    d. FDA

31. Which of the following statements concerning communications with medical direction is true?
    a. Medical direction may be at the receiving facility or at a remote site
    b. After receiving an order for a medication or procedure the communication is complete
    c. Orders that are unclear should not be carried out until arrival at the receiving facility
    d. Reports to medical direction before arrival should be lengthy so they are aware of all details
32. Which of the following statements is true concerning talking on a radio?
    a. Speak with the microphone 6 inches from your mouth
    b. Speak rapidly to minimize air time
    c. Use clear everyday language instead of codes
    d. Use simple words like "yes" and "no" instead of "affirmative" and "negative" in your discussion
33. A repeater is:
    a. A stationary radio with superior transmission and receiving capabilities
    b. A remote receiver that receives a transmission and transmits it at a higher power
    c. A digital radio that blocks out radio transmissions
    d. The console that a dispatcher uses for communication
34. EMT–Basics should notify dispatch:
    a. With information regarding the assessment findings
    b. Of arrival at the receiving facility after giving a bedside report to the staff
    c. When leaving the scene
    d. To relay patient information to medical direction
35. Which of the following is administrative information obtained for documentation?
    a. Any medications administered to the patient
    b. Time of arrival at patient
    c. Patient's chief complaint
    d. Equipment used at the scene
36. All of the following are components of the minimum data set for patient information **EXCEPT**:
    a. Type of location
    b. Patient's age and gender
    c. Chief complaint
    d. Response to treatment
37. The prehospital care report:
    a. Should contain objective and subjective information
    b. Should not be released for billing purposes
    c. Can be used for case review if patient confidentiality is protected
    d. Should include the EMT–Basic's diagnosis of the patient
38. Which of the following medical abbreviations is correct?
    a. Penicillin = Penn
    b. Chief complaint = ChCo
    c. Nothing by mouth = NPO
    d. Every = EV
39. Which of the following is true regarding documentation?
    a. Completely scratch out errors in documentation and write the correct information beside the scratched out information
    b. Document a patient's refusal of care and have your partner sign as a witness
    c. Always document the care that you wished to give, whether it was given or not
    d. Document situations such as infectious disease exposure on a special report form, submitted in a timely manner

MEDICAL/BEHAVIORAL EMERGENCIES AND OBSTETRICS AND GYNECOLOGY

CHAPTER 16
GENERAL PHARMACOLOGY

● **CHAPTER OUTLINE**

I. Medication Information

    A. Types of Medication

    B. Medication Names

    C. Medication Forms

II. Medication Administration

    A. Indications and Contraindications

    B. Administration Routes

III. Medication Actions

    A. Actions

    B. Side Effects

    C. Reassessment Strategies

● MATCHING

Match the terms in Column 1 with the correct definition in Column 2:

Column 1

1. _____ Contraindication

2. _____ Dose

3. _____ Drug

4. _____ Generic name

5. _____ Indication

6. _____ Inhalation

7. _____ Mechanism of action

8. _____ Pharmacology

9. _____ Route of administration

10. _____ Sublingual route

11. _____ Trade name

Column 2

a. route of administration for medications in the form of a fine mist or a gas

b. condition for which a medication may be used

c. science of drugs and study of their origin, ingredients, uses, and actions of the body

d. amount of medication that should be administered

e. putting a medication under the patient's tongue

f. any substance that alters the body's functioning when taken into the body

g. how a medication affects the body

h. situation in which a medication should not be used

i. name assigned by the company that sells a medication

j. way the medication is administered to the patient

k. name of a medication listed in the *U.S. Pharmacopeia,* the official name assigned to the medication

● REVIEW QUESTIONS

1. Medication and pharmacology are interchangeable terms. **True or false?**

2. EMT–Basic units carry the medications _____, _____, and _____ on the EMS unit for administration when advised by medical direction.

3. When a medication is manufactured and ready for marketing, the manufacturer gives it a _____ name.
   a. Trade
   b. Generic
   c. Common
   d. Drug

4. Medications can have more than one trade name but only one generic name. **True or false?**

5. List three forms of medications:

   a. _____

   b. _____

   c. _____

6. Match the generic name in Column 1 with the trade name in Column 2:

	Column 1	Column 2
1. _____	Oral glucose	a. Proventil
		b. Actidose
2. _____	Activated charcoal	c. Glutose
		d. Nitrostat
3. _____	Nitroglycerin	
4. _____	Albuterol	

7. A contraindication is a factor that prohibits the use of a medication or a procedure. **True or false?**

8. The dose of a medication may depend on _____.
   a. Age   c. Race
   b. Gender   d. Height

9. Oral medications can be administered to both responsive or unresponsive patients. **True or false?**

10. When drugs are administered sublingually, the medication is rapidly absorbed by _____.
    a. The vessels in the cheek   c. The digestive tract
    b. Capillaries under the tongue   d. Capillaries in the lung

11. The epinephrine autoinjector delivers medication via the _____ route.
    a. Oral   c. Inhalation
    b. Sublingual   d. Intramuscular

12. The undesirable actions of a medication are called _____

    _____.

13. Many medications have predictable side effects. **True or false?**

14. After administering a medication, carefully monitor the patient for

    _____ _____ and _____

    _____ of the drug, as well as completing ongoing assessments.

15. It is the beginning of your work shift, and you are checking out the supplies and equipment in the ambulance.
    a. What medications would you find in the ambulance?

    _____

    _____

    b. What physician-prescribed medications can you assist patients to administer?

    _____

    _____

    c. Define the terms *indication, contraindication,* and *dose.*

    _____

    _____

CHAPTER 17

RESPIRATORY EMERGENCIES

● **CHAPTER OUTLINE**

I. Respiratory System Review

    A. Anatomy

    B. Physiology

II. Breathing Assessment

    A. Adequate Breathing

    B. Breathing Difficulty

    C. Focused History and Physical Examination

III. Emergency Medical Care

    A. Oxygen

    B. Position and Transport

    C. Artificial Ventilation

    D. Inhalers

● REVIEW QUESTIONS

1. Label Figure 17-1 with the following respiratory structures:

   left bronchus   oropharynx
   nasopharynx   right bronchus
   epiglottis   larynx
   trachea   pharynx
   diaphragm

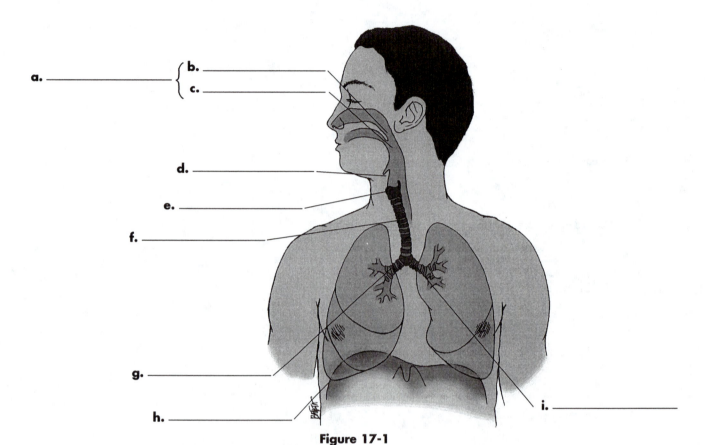

Figure 17-1

2. The exchange of oxygen and carbon dioxide occurs in the alveoli. **True or false?**

3. Inhaled air contains high concentrations of _____, whereas exhaled air contains high concentrations of _____.
   a. Oxygen; carbon dioxide   **c.** Carbon dioxide; oxygen
   b. Air; oxygen   **d.** Oxygen; air

4. What is the normal respiratory rate for a child?
   a. 25-50 breaths per minute   **c.** 15-30 breaths per minute
   b. 12-20 breaths per minute   **d.** 20-40 breaths per minute

5. Adequate breathing means the patient has a normal rate, rhythm,

   _____, and _____.

6. Inadequate breathing can occur when a patient's rate is too fast or too slow. **True or false?**

7. Changes in the rate, volume, or quality of breathing affects the amount of

   _____ available to the cells.

8. Indicate which of the following is **NOT** a sign or symptom of respiratory distress:
   a. Shortness of breath   **c.** Shallow respirations
   b. Rapid respiratory rate   **d.** Speaking in full sentences

9. It is not unusual for respirations to be noisy. **True or false?**

10. List at least three signs and symptoms of difficulty breathing in each of the following categories:

    General

    a. _____

    b. _____

    c. _____

    Visual

    a. _____

    b. _____

    c. _____

    Auditory

    a. _____

    b. _____

    c. _____

11. A barrel chest may indicate a long history of respiratory problems. **True or false?**

12. Define each of the following letters from the OPQRST acronym:

    O _____

    P _____

    Q _____

    R _____

    S _____

    T _____

13. Patients with difficulty breathing should be transported lying flat to maximize their breathing effort. **True or false?**

14. The first medication to administer to a patient in respiratory distress is

    _____.

15. An inhaler is a medication that is carried by EMTs on the EMS unit. **True or false?**

16. A beta-agonist inhaler is used to _____ bronchioles and _____ resistance inside airways.
    a. Dilate; increase   c. Restrict; increase
    b. Dilate; decrease   d. Restrict; decrease

17. Albuterol and isoetharine are _____ names for the medication in an inhaler.

18. List three criteria for the use of an inhaler:

    a. _____

    b. _____

    c. _____

19. List at least three contraindications for the use of a prescribed inhaler.

    a. _____

    b. _____

    c. _____

20. The spacer should be removed from an inhaler before administration. **True or false?**

21. Patients of any age can use an inhaler. **True or false?**

22. Which of the following is a possible side effect from an inhaler.
    a. Increased heart rate   c. Decreased blood pressure
    b. Altered mental status   d. Cyanosis

23. Number the following steps for assisting with a prescribed inhaler in the proper order, with 1 as the first step and 6 as the last:

    _____ Hold breath as long as comfortable

    _____ Check expiration date

    _____ Remove oxygen mask, patient exhales deeply

    _____ Shake vigorously

    _____ Begin inhalation, depress inhaler

    _____ Place mouth over inhaler mouthpiece

24. You have been dispatched to a funeral home where a grieving widow is having difficulty breathing. On your arrival, you find a 46-year-old woman sitting in the lobby surrounded by family. Her daughter tells you that the breathing problem came on suddenly and that her mother "can't seem to catch her breath."
    a. What are the general signs and symptoms of difficulty breathing?

    _____

    _____

    _____

    b. As your partner applies high-concentration oxygen, what information should you obtain from the patient or family?

    _____

    _____

    _____

    c. The patient has no significant medical history, does not take any medications, and has vital signs within normal limits. She agrees to be transported to the hospital for physician evaluation. How will you position this patient for transport?

    _____

    _____

    _____

25. You have responded to an elementary school where a 10-year-old student is having a possible asthma attack. On arrival, you find the child and his teacher sitting inside the entryway of the school. The boy is in moderate distress and has audible wheezing. He is holding a metered-dose inhaler in his hand.

a. What are common trade names for bronchodilators?

_____

_____

_____

b. How do bronchodilators work to decrease resistance inside the airways?

_____

_____

_____

c. What information should you obtain from this patient before contacting medical direction?

_____

_____

_____

d. What are the three criteria that must be met before assisting this patient with his medication?

_____

_____

_____

CHAPTER 18

CARDIOVASCULAR EMERGENCIES

● **CHAPTER OUTLINE**

I. Review of the Circulatory System

    A. Anatomy

        1. Blood vessels

        2. Blood composition

    B. Physiology

II. Cardiac Compromise

    A. Assessment

    B. Emergency Medical Care

        1. Oxygen and positioning

        2. Nitroglycerin

        3. Basic life support

III. The Automated External Defibrillator

    A. Overview of the Automated External Defibrillator

    B. Advantages of the Automated External Defibrillator

    C. Operation of the Automated External Defibrillator

    D. Postresuscitation Care

    E. Automated External Defibrillator Maintenance

    F. Automated External Defibrillator Skills

● MATCHING

Match the terms in column 1 with the correct definition in Column 2:

Column 1

1. _____ Angina

2. _____ Diastolic blood pressure

3. _____ Electrodes

4. _____ Ischemia

5. _____ Peripheral

6. _____ Pulse

7. _____ Systolic blood pressure

8. _____ Ventricular fibrillation

9. _____ Ventricular tachycardia

Column 2

a. remote pads attached to the defibrillator and the patient to monitor the electrical activity of the heart

b. decreased oxygen supply to an area of tissue

c. chaotic electrical rhythm in the ventricles, with no contraction of the ventricles and no pulse

d. measurement of the pressure in an artery when the ventricles are contracting

e. three or more heart beats in a row at 100 beats or more per minute originating in the ventricles

f. measurement of the pressure in an artery when the ventricles are at rest

g. term referring to the extremities

h. pressure wave felt in an artery when the left ventricle contracts

i. discomfort felt when the heart does not receive enough oxygen

10. Using arrows, indicate the blood flow through the heart on Figure 18-1.

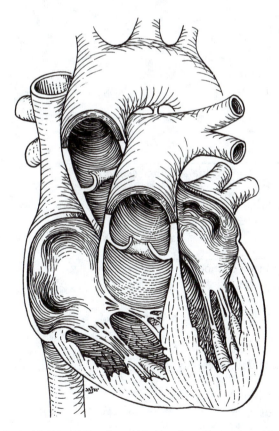

Figure 18-1 From McKenna/Sanders: *Workbook to Accompany Mosby's Paramedic Textbook*, 1994, Mosby Lifeline.

● REVIEW QUESTIONS

1. The heart consists of four chambers with valves between them that work together to circulate blood to the lungs and body. **True or false?**

2. Match the arteries in Column 1 with the correct location in Column 2:

Column 1	Column 2
1. _____ Iliac	**a.** foot
	b. groin
2. _____ Coronary	**c.** heart
	d. lungs
3. _____ Pulmonary	**e.** pelvis
	f. arm
4. _____ Carotid	**g.** wrist
	h. neck
5. _____ Brachial	
6. _____ Femoral	
7. _____ Radial	
8. _____ Dorsalis pedis	

3. Blood from the vena cavae enters the _____.
   a. Right atrium   **c.** Left ventricle
   b. Left atrium   **d.** Right ventricle

4. Blood contains plasma, red cells, white cells, and _____.

5. A pulse should be generated every time the left ventricle contracts. **True or false?**

6. List two sites for locating central pulses and two sites for locating peripheral pulses.

   Central   Peripheral

   a. _____   **b.** _____

   _____   _____

7. The first number in a blood pressure is the _____ value and the second number is the _____ value.
   a. Systolic; contracting   **c.** Systolic; diastolic
   b. Diastolic; resting   **d.** None of the above

8. Another term used to describe shock is _____.

9. Which of the following is **NOT** a sign or symptom of shock?
   a. Rapid, weak pulse   **c.** Cool, clammy skin
   b. High blood pressure   **d.** Anxiety

10. Chest pressure or discomfort that usually goes away with rest is called

    _____.

11. In a heart attack, a blood vessel is blocked and the heart muscle can no longer get _____. This is called _____.
    a. Blood; angina   **c.** White cells; ischemia
    b. Oxygen; ischemia   **d.** Oxygen; tissue damage

12. Respiratory pain is often _____ and _____ with breathing. Cardiac pain is usually _____ and _____ with movement.

13. List at least three locations where cardiac pain may radiate.

   a. _____

   b. _____

   c. _____

14. Severity can be measured on a scale of 1 to 10 where 10 is the _____ pain.

15. Define each of the following components of the OPQRST acronym.

   O _____

   P _____

   Q _____

   R _____

   S _____

   T _____

16. The first medication delivered to the cardiac patient is _____.

17. How would you transport a responsive patient with no trauma, complaining of chest pain?
   a. Sitting up   c. Recovery position
   b. Lying down   d. Position of comfort

18. If the patient has nitroglycerin you should administer it prior to beginning your assessment. **True or false?**

19. Nitroglycerin acts by _____ blood vessels, which may _____ blood pressure.
   a. Constricting; decrease   c. Dilating; increase
   b. Dilating; decrease   d. Constricting; increase

20. List at least three contraindications for nitroglycerin.

   a. _____

   b. _____

   c. _____

21. All of the following are common side effects of nitroglycerin EXCEPT:
   a. Muscle tremors   c. Lowered blood pressure
   b. Headache   d. Burning sensation under the tongue

22. The primary intervention that makes the most difference in survival from cardiac arrest is _____.

23. The term used to describe a quivering heart muscle is _____.
   a. Cardiac arrest   c. Ventricular fibrillation
   b. Defibrillation   d. None of the above

24. Before placement of an AED the EMT must confirm that the patient is

_____, _____, and

_____.

    a. Pulseless; breathing; unresponsive
    b. Pulseless; breathing; responsive
    c. Pulseless; not breathing; unresponsive
    d. Breathing; with a pulse; has chest pain

25. Coming in contact with the patient or stretcher during defibrillation could result in a shock or burn. **True or false?**

26. CPR may be stopped for up to _____ to allow delivery of three stacked shocks from the AED.

    a. 30 seconds   **c.** 90 seconds
    b. 1 minute   **d.** 2 minutes

27. A patient must weigh at least _____ pounds and

be at least _____ years of age before the AED can be used.

28. The maximum number of shocks that should be delivered before initiating transport is _____.

    a. 6   **c.** 9
    b. 3   **d.** 12

29. Each shock should be followed by two ventilations and a pulse check. **True or false?**

30. You are caring for a 76-year-old man who is complaining of chest pain. The pain began about 30 minutes ago when he was taking his morning walk. He took one nitroglycerin tablet before your arrival. Using a severity scale of 1 to 10, the patient rated his pain as an 8 when it started. After resting and taking a nitroglycerin tablet, he says it is now a 6. You administer high-concentration oxygen by mask and obtain a set of vitals. His blood pressure is 166/84, pulse is 122 and regular, and respirations are 16. The patient looks anxious and is slightly diaphoretic.

    a. Describe angina.

_____

_____

_____

    b. What are the three indications for nitroglycerin administration?

_____

_____

_____

    c. What are the five contraindications for nitroglycerin administration?

_____

_____

_____

31. It is 0300, and your crew has been dispatched for a "possible heart attack." On arrival, you find a 52-year-old woman sitting on a sofa in her living room. She tells you that her chest pain woke her from sleep about an hour ago and has not "let up." Your partner applies high-concentration oxygen and obtains a set of vital signs while you gather a SAMPLE history. Her vitals are within normal range, and she has no significant medical history.

  a. What are common signs and symptoms of cardiac compromise?

  _____

  _____

  b. As you prepare the patient for transport, she tells you that she has some nitroglycerin tablets that belong to a friend. Can you assist her in taking this medication?

  _____

  _____

32. Your crew has been dispatched to a possible drug overdose at a local high school. On arrival, you are directed to the gym where you find a 17-year-old student lying on the floor. The coach tells you that the student was acting "a little strange" just before he collapsed. You position the patient supine, open his airway, and assess breathing and circulation. The student is breathless and pulseless. You initiate CPR, attach the AED, and request ALS back-up.

  a. What two rhythms will the AED recognize as shockable rhythms?

  _____

  _____

  b. Describe proper placement of the AED electrodes.

  _____

  _____

  c. If a shockable rhythm is identified by the AED, how many shocks will be delivered in one cycle?

  _____

  _____

  d. What is the energy level of each shock?

  _____

  _____

CHAPTER 19

DIABETES AND ALTERED MENTAL STATUS

● **CHAPTER OUTLINE**

I. Causes of Altered Mental Status

    A. Diabetic Emergency

    B. Seizures

    C. Other Possible Causes

II. Emergency Care of Patients With Altered Mental Status

    A. Assessment

    B. Airway Management

    C. Treatment for Diabetic Emergency

● MATCHING

Match the terms in Column 1 with the correct definition in Column 2:

Column 1	Column 2
1. _____ Altered mental status	**a.** low level of sugar in the blood
	b. diabetic patient who requires hormone injections for the body to use sugar
2. _____ Diabetes mellitus	
3. _____ Glucose	**c.** rapid discharge of nerve cells in the brain causing muscular contractions
4. _____ Hypoglycemia	**d.** disease that prevents insulin from being produced
5. _____ Insulin-dependent	**e.** form of sugar that is converted into usable energy
6. _____ Seizure	**f.** state of mind in which the patient is not oriented to person, place, or time (not necessarily all three together)

● REVIEW QUESTIONS

1. Altered mental status is only related to medical conditions. **True or false?**
2. List two common signs and symptoms of hypoglycemia:

   a. _____

   b. _____
3. Seizures can cause full body jerking or just blank staring into space. **True or false?**
4. List at least three common causes of seizures:

   a. _____

   b. _____

   c. _____
5. All seizures are life threatening. **True or false?**
6. One of the most common causes of seizures in children is

   _____.
7. The time following a seizure when a patient may be disoriented is called the

   _____ period.
8. List at least three common causes of altered mental status:

   a. _____

   b. _____

   c. _____
9. The primary goal of emergency treatment for patients with altered mental

   status is maintaining a(n) _____.

10. List at least three major points for the focused history and physical examination of a patient with altered mental status.

a. _____

b. _____

c. _____

11. An evaluation of the scene can be an important part of assessing a patient with altered mental status. **True or false?**

12. Patients with altered mental status are considered _____ and vital signs are monitored every _____.
   a. Stable; 5 minutes   c. Unstable; 5 minutes
   b. Unstable; 15 minutes   d. Stable; 15 minutes

13. List two questions to ask a patient with altered mental status and a history of diabetes:

a. _____

b. _____

14. Oral glucose should be used for all patients with altered mental status. **True or false?**

15. Oral glucose should be used only if the patient can swallow. **True or false?**

16. Oral glucose is the product's _____ name.
   a. Generic   c. Chemical
   b. Trade   d. Brand

17. To administer oral glucose, squirt the tube into the mouth and let the patient swallow. **True or false?**

18. Absence of a _____ _____ is a contraindication for administration of oral glucose.

19. Oral glucose improves the patient's condition by increasing

_____ _____.

20. Medical direction must be involved in the decision to administer oral glucose. **True or false?**

21. You and your partner have had an unusually busy shift. You know that she has insulin-controlled diabetes, and you are concerned because you have missed both breakfast and lunch. Just as you are about to grab a bite to eat, you are dispatched to a car crash.
   a. What type of diabetic reaction might your partner experience and why?

_____

_____

_____

b. What are common signs and symptoms of a diabetic emergency?

_____

_____

_____

c. En route to the scene, your partner eats a candy bar from her purse. If her condition had progressed to an altered mental status, how would you manage this situation?

_____

_____

_____

22. Your crew has been dispatched to a possible cardiac arrest. On arrival, you find a man in his mid-twenties lying face down on the ground. A passerby found the man in this condition and dialed 9-1-1 on his cellular phone. No patient information is available.
   a. What are your first priorities of care for this patient?

_____

_____

   b. The patient is breathing but is unresponsive to verbal or painful stimuli. You control his airway and administer high-concentration oxygen. What common causes of altered mental status should you consider?

_____

_____

   c. How will you manage this patient?

_____

_____

CHAPTER 20

ALLERGIC REACTIONS

● **CHAPTER OUTLINE**

    I. Assessment of Allergic Reactions

        A. Causes of Allergic Reactions

        B. Signs and Symptoms of Allergic Reactions

    II. Emergency Care for Patients With Allergic Reactions

        A. Airway Management

        B. Administration of Medication

● REVIEW QUESTIONS

1. An allergic reaction can best be described as:
   a. A life-threatening emergency
   b. A normal response to an allergen
   c. High blood pressure following a reaction
   d. An exaggerated response to an allergen

2. Allergic reactions are always life threatening and must be treated immediately. **True or false?**

3. List three common allergens:

   a. _____

   b. _____

   c. _____

4. List five common signs and symptoms of an allergic reaction:

   a. _____

   b. _____

   c. _____

   d. _____

   e. _____

5. Itchy, watery eyes, runny nose, and a headache are all signs and symptoms

   of a _____ allergic reaction.

6. The first sign of hypoperfusion may be a change in _____

   _____ _____.

7. In an allergic reaction, an altered mental status is caused by decreased

   _____ to the tissues.

8. A true medical emergency exists when the patient shows signs or symptoms
   of _____ or _____.
   a. Hypoperfusion; high blood pressure
   b. Hypoperfusion; respiratory compromise
   c. Respiratory compromise; nausea
   d. Headache; feeling of doom

9. Epinephrine autoinjectors are used only on patients with signs and symptoms
   of _____ and _____.
   a. Hypoperfusion; high blood pressure
   b. Hypoperfusion; respiratory compromise
   c. Respiratory compromise; nausea
   d. Headache; feeling of doom

10. A patient with an allergic reaction and signs of respiratory compromise

    should be assessed at least every _____ minutes.

11. Epinephrine works by _____ bronchioles and _____ blood vessels.
    a. Dilating; constricting   c. Constricting; constricting
    b. Dilating; dilating   d. Constricting; dilating

12. List the three criteria for use of the epinephrine autoinjector:

   a. _____

   b. _____

   c. _____

13. There are several contraindications for the EMT–Basic administering an epi-nephrine autoinjector for a patient with life-threatening airway compromise. **True or false?**

14. An autoinjector consists of a needle and syringe of medication, which is injected when pressed against the skin. **True or false?**

15. Which of the following is **NOT** a side effect of epinephrine:
   a. Dizziness   c. Sleepiness
   b. Pale skin   d. Nausea and vomiting

16. Airway control is secondary to using the autoinjector in a patient having an allergic reaction. **True or false?**

17. You have been dispatched to a public swimming pool at the city park. On arrival, you find a 36-year-old man who says he has been stung by a bee. He is near hysterics and tells you that he is highly allergic to stings. He has an epinephrine autoinjector in his bag but is afraid to inject himself.
   a. What are common signs and symptoms of an allergic reaction?

   _____

   _____

   b. The patient has several of the signs and symptoms of an allergic reaction and is complaining of difficulty breathing. What are the criteria for use of an epinephrine autoinjector?

   _____

   _____

   c. Medical direction authorizes you to administer the epinephrine. Describe the steps in drug administration.

   _____

   _____

18. You are working during part of your vacation as a counselor at a youth camp. The administrator knows that you are an EMT–Basic and asks you to look at a child who is feeling sick. The 9-year-old girl is complaining of itchy, watery eyes and has a runny nose and a headache. As you examine her, you notice a rash on her neck and abdomen. Her vital signs are within normal limits and her lung sounds are clear. The child tells you that she is allergic to "a lot of things" but has no medications.
   a. What are common causes of mild allergic reactions?

   _____

   _____

b. What assessment findings would reveal a severe allergic reaction in this patient?

_____

_____

c. Would this patient be a candidate for epinephrine administration? Why or why not?

_____

_____

CHAPTER 21

POISONING AND OVERDOSE

● **CHAPTER OUTLINE**

  I. History of Poisoning

  II. Types of Toxins

    A. Ingested Toxins

    B. Inhaled Toxins

    C. Injected Toxins

    D. Absorbed Toxins

  III. Airway Management

  IV. Use of Activated Charcoal

● MATCHING

Match the terms in Column 1 with the correct definition in Column 2:

Column 1	Column 2
1. _____ Absorbed toxin	**a.** substance that produces adverse effects when it enters the body
2. _____ Activated charcoal	**b.** toxin that enters the body through a puncture in the skin
3. _____ Ingested toxin	**c.** toxin that enters the body through the skin
4. _____ Inhaled toxin	**d.** toxin that is consumed orally
	e. toxin that is breathed into the lungs where it is absorbed into the bloodstream
5. _____ Injected toxin	
6. _____ Toxin	**f.** medication that medical direction may authorize for management of poisoning caused by an ingested toxin

● REVIEW QUESTIONS

1. A larger than recommended dose of any medication can be considered a poisoning. **True or false?**

2. Ongoing assessments are every _____ minutes for

   unstable patients and every _____ minutes for stable patients.

3. List four questions to assist you in gathering information about the poisoning or overdose patient:

   a. _____

   b. _____

   c. _____

   d. _____

4. An overdose is an intentional use of too much medication. **True or false?**

5. Asking about time since exposure will _____.
   a. Provide valuable information about side effects
   b. Help determine treatment options
   c. Aid medical direction in determining source
   d. None of the above

6. Over-the-counter treatments for poisoning and overdoses are beneficial and should be encouraged. **True or false?**

7. Diarrhea and peculiar breath odors are common side effects of _____ toxins.
   a. Inhaled   c. Absorbed
   b. Ingested   d. Injected

8. If pills or tablets are still in the mouth of an unresponsive patient, how should the EMT–Basic handle the pills?

_____

_____

9. List three common signs and symptoms of inhaled toxins:

    a. _____

    b. _____

    c. _____

10. The primary treatment for inhaled poisoning is _____.
11. Localized findings of swelling, itching, and redness are signs and symptoms associated with _____ toxins.
    a. Inhaled   c. Absorbed
    b. Ingested   d. Injected
12. Injected toxins reach the body through all of the following routes **EXCEPT**:
    a. Bites   c. Stings
    b. IV   d. Sublingual
13. Always bring the possible toxin to the receiving facility. **True or false?**
14. The rate of absorption for injected toxic material is affected by all of the following **EXCEPT**:
    a. Location of injection site   c. Blood flow to area
    b. Gender of the patient   d. Type of animal
15. Powder or liquid on the skin may result in an _____ toxin.
    a. Inhaled   c. Absorbed
    b. Ingested   d. Injected
16. Dry substances should be _____ away and liquid substances _____ away.
    a. Brushed; irrigated   c. Blown; wiped
    b. Irrigated; irrigated   d. Irrigated; blotted
17. Activated charcoal is the treatment for _____ toxins.
    a. Inhaled   c. Absorbed
    b. Ingested   d. Injected

18. Activated charcoal works by _____ to the toxin in the

    _____.
19. Activated charcoal is the _____ name. LiquiChar and InstaChar are _____ names.
    a. Generic; trade   c. Chemical; trade
    b. Trade; generic   d. Brand; generic
20. List three contraindications for the use of activated charcoal:

    a. _____

    b. _____

    c. _____
21. Vomiting is a desired effect of administration of activated charcoal. **True or false?**

22. You have been dispatched to care for a 4-year-old child who has ingested an unknown amount of baby aspirin. On arrival, you find the mother holding the child in her lap. The child appears anxious but is not in obvious distress. The mother tells you that she found the child playing with two empty aspirin bottles about 20 minutes ago. She does not know how many pills were in the bottles. You contact medical direction and give your patient report. The physician advises you to administer activated charcoal.

   a. What is the normal dose of activated charcoal for infants and children?

   _____

   _____

   b. What are the indications and contraindications for administering activated charcoal?

   _____

   _____

   c. You administer the activated charcoal as directed. En route to the hospital, the patient vomits. What should you do?

   _____

   _____

23. You are caring for a patient who has attempted suicide. He was found in his car by a neighbor who noticed the car's engine was running while the garage door was closed. You and your partner move the patient outside and perform an initial assessment of his airway, breathing, and circulation. He is unresponsive and has a pulse and shallow respirations at six per minute.

   a. What treatment is indicated first for this patient?

   _____

   _____

   b. Describe the characteristics of carbon monoxide and the general symptoms of exposure.

   _____

   _____

   c. In what other scenario is carbon monoxide commonly present?

   _____

   _____

CHAPTER 22
ENVIRONMENTAL EMERGENCIES

● **CHAPTER OUTLINE**

I. Thermoregulatory Emergencies

    A. Temperature Regulation in the Body

    B. Exposure to the Cold

        1. Generalized hypothermia

            a. Predisposing factors

            b. Signs and symptoms of generalized hypothermia

            c. Emergency care for patients with generalized hypothermia

        2. Local cold injuries

            a. Predisposing factors

            b. Signs and symptoms of local cold injuries

            c. Emergency care for patients with local cold injuries

    C. Exposure to Heat

        1. Predisposing factors

        2. Signs and symptoms of generalized hyperthermia

        3. Emergency care for patients with generalized hyperthermia

II. Drowning and Near Drowning

    A. Emergency Medical Care of the Near-Drowning Patient

III. Bites and Stings

    A. Signs and Symptoms

    B. Emergency Medical Care for Bites and Stings

● MATCHING

Match the terms in Column 1 with the correct definition in Column 2:

	Column 1		Column 2
1. _____	Conduction	a.	any condition involving a significant change in temperature of the body
2. _____	Convection	b.	condition in which the body temperature is above normal (98.6° F or 38° C)
3. _____	Evaporation		
4. _____	Hyperthermia	c.	loss of heat, in the form of infrared energy, to cooler surroundings
		d.	transfer of heat directly from one object to another
5. _____	Hypothermia	e.	transfer of heat to moving air or liquid
6. _____	Radiation		
		f.	transfer of heat that occurs when a liquid changes into a gas
7. _____	Thermoregulatory emergency	g.	condition in which the body temperature is below normal (98.6° F or 37° C)

● REVIEW QUESTIONS

1. The temperature of the body needs to remain fairly constant to maintain vital chemical functions. **True or false?**

2. The human body loses heat by evaporation, conduction, radiation,

   _____, and _____.

3. When body temperature begins to decrease, the body produces heat by

   _____.

4. When body temperature begins to increase, the body produces

   _____, which cools the body by evaporation.

5. Any time the body temperature drops below normal the patient is hypothermic. **True or false?**

6. The most common cause of generalized hypothermia is submersion in water. **True or false?**

7. List at least five predisposing factors for generalized hypothermia:

   a. _____

   b. _____

   c. _____

   d. _____

   e. _____

8. An unreliable sign of hypothermia is cool _____.

9. Cool _____ _____ is a sign of a generalized cold emergency.

10. All of the following are signs and symptoms of early hypothermia **EXCEPT:**
    - **a.** Shivering
    - **c.** Slow respirations
    - **b.** Rapid pulse
    - **d.** Normal blood pressure
11. A rapid pulse and respirations are the body's attempt to increase heat production. **True or false?**
12. Define active rewarming and passive rewarming:

    Active rewarming-
    _____

    _____

    Passive rewarming-
    _____

    _____

13. Heat packs at the axillae and groin are a form of _____ rewarming.
14. Active rewarming is a vital part of treatment for the patient in late hypothermia with decreased level of responsiveness. **True or false?**
15. A pulse check for a severely hypothermic patient should be between

    _____ and _____ seconds.
16. List five body areas most susceptible to localized cold injuries:

    a. _____

    b. _____

    c. _____

    d. _____

    e. _____

17. Which of the following is **NOT** a sign or symptom of late, localized cold damage?
    - **a.** Waxy or white skin
    - **c.** Tingling sensation
    - **b.** Swelling, blisters
    - **d.** Firm feeling when touched
18. Rubbing and massaging a cold injury is beneficial because it causes blood flow to return to the area. **True or false?**
19. List four predisposing factors for heat emergencies:

    a. _____

    b. _____

    c. _____

    d. _____

20. Hot skin is a late sign of an extreme heat emergency. **True or false?**
21. Care for the patient with generalized hyperthermia and hot skin include:
    - **a.** Fan the patient and turn up air conditioning
    - **b.** Keep the skin wet
    - **c.** Apply cool packs to the underarms and in groin
    - **d.** All of the above

22. Define drowning and near drowning:

_____

_____

_____

23. Patients found unresponsive in the water should be treated and evaluated

for possible _____ injury.

24. Bites and stings may cause localized reactions but also may produce a(n)

_____ reaction.

25. The first priority in a bite or sting emergency is to remove the stinger from the patient. **True or false?**

26. For an extremity bite or sting, position the injured area _____.
   a. At heart level
   b. Below heart level
   c. Above heart level
   d. Positioning of the extremity is not important

27. Credit cards or rigid cardboard can be used to scrape out a stinger. **True or false?**

28. You have been dispatched to a nearby ski resort to care for an accident victim. On arrival, you find a 30-year-old woman who was injured on one of the ski slopes. Her friends had reported her missing for several hours. She was rescued and brought to the lodge by members of the ski patrol. She has an injury to her right lower extremity and appears to be suffering from hypothermia.
   a. What are the predisposing factors for generalized hypothermia?

_____

_____

_____

   b. What mental status and motor function changes may be caused by hypothermia?

_____

_____

_____

   c. What are general principles for treating all hypothermic patients?

_____

_____

_____

29. Your crew has been dispatched to standby at a rescue operation where a car has been submerged in a lake. Shortly after your arrival, one of the divers becomes trapped beneath the water. While trying to free himself, his air hose is cut by the car's wreckage. He is brought to the surface by other members of the rescue team. He is unresponsive and in respiratory arrest.

a. What are your first priorities in managing this patient?

_____

_____

b. During resuscitation, the patient's abdomen swells and begins to interfere with ventilation. What should you do?

_____

_____

c. Should attempts always be made to relieve gastric distention in victims of near drowning? Why or why not?

_____

_____

CHAPTER 23

BEHAVIORAL EMERGENCIES

● **CHAPTER OUTLINE**

I. Behavior

    A. Behavioral Changes

    B. Psychologic Crises

    C. Suicidal Gestures

II. Assessment and Emergency Care

    A. Scene Size-up

    B. Communication and Emergency Medical Care

    C. Calming the Patient

    D. Restraints

III. Medical and Legal Considerations

    A. Consent

    B. Resistance to Treatment

    C. Use of Force

    D. Documentation

● MATCHING

Match the terms in Column 1 with the correct definition in Column 2:

Column 1	Column 2
1. _____ Abnormal behavior	a. form of violence that results from a family argument and may result in abuse of spouse or children
2. _____ Behavioral emergency	b. refers to behavior by a person who has lost touch with reality
3. _____ Domestic dispute	c. power necessary to keep a person from injuring him/herself or others
4. _____ Psychotic	d. actions exhibited by a person that is outside of the norm for the situation and is socially unacceptable
5. _____ Reasonable force	e. situation in which a person acts in a manner that is unacceptable or intolerable to the person, family members, or the community

● REVIEW QUESTIONS

1. The way in which people act on a day-to-day basis is called their

   _____.

2. List three factors that can alter a person's behavior:

   a. _____

   b. _____

   c. _____

3. Patients experiencing psychotic thinking should be treated _____.
   a. As any other patient
   c. Loudly to get their attention
   b. Carefully and calmly
   d. None of the above

4. List three risk factors associated with suicide:

   a. _____

   b. _____

   c. _____

5. Suicidal patients will demonstrate at least one risk factor. **True or false?**

6. The scene size-up is the most important part of entering a scene with a potential behavioral emergency. **True or false?**

7. Which of the following is **NOT** a sign of potential violence?
   a. Sitting back on the couch or chair, frowning
   b. Throwing things
   c. Holding a potentially dangerous object
   d. Clenched fists

8. If the patient has a history of behavioral problem he/she will not require evaluation for medical or trauma-related problems. **True or false?**

9. Avoid agreeing with patients who appear to have disturbed thinking patterns. **True or false?**

10. Patients who do not calm down or are showing signs of destructive behavior

    may need to be _____.

11. Restraints may help you provide adequate care to the patient, but if used incorrectly they can cause _____.

12. Restraints should be removed as soon as the patient begins to calm down to avoid injury. **True or false?**

13. No patient can be transported against his/her will. **True or false?**

14. List three points that must be documented for behavioral emergencies:

    a. _____

    b. _____

    c. _____

15. Assistance in determining the need for transport of a patient refusing care should be obtained through _____ _____.

16. The amount of force required to keep patients from injuring themselves or others is called _____ force.

17. Local law enforcement personnel have requested EMS to transport a patient to the hospital for psychological evaluation. You arrive at the scene and find a 30-year-old man who claims the FBI is trying to kill him. The police have placed him in protective custody and the scene is safe.

    a. What type of communication should you attempt with this patient? Provide examples of questions you should ask.

    _____

    _____

    _____

    b. What methods can you use to calm this patient?

    _____

    _____

    _____

    c. What type of documentation is considered important when caring for a patient with a behavioral emergency?

    _____

    _____

    _____

CHAPTER 24

OBSTETRICS AND GYNECOLOGY

● CHAPTER OUTLINE

I. Reproductive Anatomy and Physiology

   A. Labor

II. Contents of the Childbirth Kit

III. Predelivery Emergencies

   A. Miscarriage

      1. Emergency care for miscarriage

   B. Seizure During Pregnancy

      1. Emergency care for seizure during pregnancy

   C. Vaginal Bleeding Late in Pregnancy

      1. Emergency care for bleeding late in pregnancy

   D. Trauma

      1. Emergency care for trauma in pregnancy

IV. Normal Delivery

   A. Predelivery Considerations

   B. Precautions

   C. Delivery Procedure

   D. Initial Care of the Newborn

V. Abnormal Deliveries and Complications

    A. Prolapsed Cord

        1. Emergency care for prolapsed cord

    B. Breech Presentation

        1. Emergency care for breech presentation

    C. Limb Presentation

        1. Emergency care for limb presentation

    D. Multiple Births

        1. Emergency care for multiple births

    E. Meconium

        1. Emergency care when meconium is present

    F. Premature Birth

        1. Emergency care for premature birth

VI. Gynecologic Emergencies

    A. Vaginal Bleeding

    B. Trauma to External Genitalia

    C. Sexual Assault

● MATCHING

Match the terms in Column 1 with the correct definition in Column 2:

Column 1

1. _____ Abortion
2. _____ Amniotic sac
3. _____ Birth canal
4. _____ Bloody show
5. _____ Breech presentation
6. _____ Caesarean section
7. _____ Cephalic
8. _____ Cervix
9. _____ Crowning
10. _____ Fetus
11. _____ Meconium
12. _____ Miscarriage
13. _____ Perineum
14. _____ Placenta
15. _____ Presenting part
16. _____ Prolapsed cord
17. _____ Umbilical cord
18. _____ Uterus
19. _____ Vagina

Column 2

a. connects the placenta to the fetus
b. presentation of the baby's feet or buttocks first in delivery
c. the canal that leads from the uterus to the external opening in women
d. the lower part of the uterus and the vagina
e. membrane forming a closed, fluid-filled pouch around a developing fetus
f. fetal and maternal organ through which the fetus absorbs oxygen and nutrients and excretes wastes
g. stage in which the head of the baby is seen at the vaginal opening
h. situation in which the umbilical cord delivers through the vagina before any presenting part
i. presentation of baby's head first in delivery
j. area of skin between the vagina and anus
k. expulsion of the mucous plug as the cervix dilates
l. neck of the uterus
m. an unborn, developing baby
n. spontaneous delivery of a human fetus before it is able to live on its own
o. medical term for any delivery or removal of a human fetus before it can live on its own
p. fetal stool that may be present in the amniotic fluid
q. area of the fetus that appears at the vaginal opening first
r. female reproductive organ in which a baby grows and develops
s. surgical delivery in which the muscles of the abdomen are cut and the baby is delivered through the abdomen

● REVIEW QUESTIONS

1. The fetus grows and develops in the _____.
2. During pregnancy the fetus receives nutrition from the mother through the

_____.
3. The placenta is always present in a woman's uterus but is only used during pregnancy. **True or false?**
4. The fetus rests in a sac filled with 1 to 2 L of _____.
   a. Blood   c. Amniotic fluid
   b. Water   d. Plasma

5. The usual length of a pregnancy is _____ or _____.
   a. 6 months; 40 weeks   c. 9 months; 36 weeks
   b. 9 months; 40 weeks   d. 8 months; 36 weeks

6. During pregnancy a woman's blood volume _____ to accommodate for the needs of the baby.

7. The delivery of the baby ends the second stage of labor. **True or false?**

8. Crowning is a sign that delivery is about 30 to 45 minutes away. **True or false?**

9. List three pieces of equipment in the OB kit and how they are used:

   a. _____

   b. _____

   c. _____

10. The care for a woman who is experiencing a predelivery is the same as for any patient exhibiting similar signs and symptoms. **True or false?**

11. Labor pains are associated with the contraction of the _____.

12. Personal protective equipment needed during a delivery is usually limited to gloves. **True or false?**

13. A miscarriage usually occurs in the first _____ months of a pregnancy.

14. List three of the questions that will be important to ask to determine if there is enough time to transport the patient before delivery of the baby:

   a. _____

   b. _____

   c. _____

15. How would you prepare the mother for delivery?

   _____

   _____

16. Apply gentle pressure to the _____ to prevent a rapid or explosive delivery.
   a. Head of the fetus   c. Vagina
   b. Perineum   d. Abdomen

17. As the infant's head is delivered, check the neck for the presence of the _____.
   a. Umbilical cord   c. Tissue
   b. Placenta   d. None of the above

18. Suction the baby's mouth and nose with a _____ prior to delivery of the torso.

19. The umbilical cord should be cut:
   a. After pulsations stop in the cord
   b. Immediately after the baby delivers
   c. Before the placenta delivers
   d. At the receiving facility

20. After the baby delivers, gently pull on the umbilical cord until the placenta delivers. **True or false?**

21. The placenta should be wrapped and discarded prior to transport of the mother and infant. **True or false?**

22. If the mother loses more than 500 mL of blood during the delivery, the EMT–

    Basic should provide _____ _____.

23. Which of the following is **NOT** part of the initial and ongoing assessment of the newborn?
    a. Appearance   **d.** Respiratory effort
    b. Smile   **e.** Activity
    c. Pulse

24. The heart rate of a newborn should be greater than _____
    beats per minute.

25. A newborn baby has slow and shallow respirations, and the EMT–Basic provides ventilations at 60 per minute with a BVM. The heart rate is 68. The EMT–Basic should:
    a. Provide free-flow oxygen
    b. Flick the soles of the baby's feet
    c. Provide chest compressions along with ventilation
    d. Continue with BVM ventilations only

26. To transport a patient with prolapsed cord _____.
    a. Turn her on her side and transport
    b. Elevate her hips or place her in a head-down position
    c. Lay her on her stomach
    d. None of the above

27. To prevent suffocation during a breech presentation, _____.
    a. With a gloved hand, form a "V" around the baby's face
    b. Rotate the baby to be face up
    c. Pull gently on the baby until it delivers
    d. Nothing can be done

28. Which of the following statements is true concerning multiple births:
    a. Babies from multiple births are often smaller and premature
    b. Mothers will always know they are having twins
    c. Complications are not common with multiple births
    d. Cut the umbilical cords only after both babies have been born

29. A limb presentation is a true emergency and the mother should be transported immediately. **True or false?**

30. Meconium in the amniotic fluid may present a respiratory problem for a newborn. **True or false?**

31. Infants born at less than 28 weeks, or 7 months, are considered to be

    _____.

32. Resuscitation, including CPR, is more likely to be required for a premature infant as opposed to a full-term infant. **True or false?**

33. Discourage a sexual assault patient from bathing or cleaning until after evaluation at the receiving facility. **True or false?**

34. Your crew is dispatched to an "OB case." En route, you are advised that the patient is full term and that her water has broken. On arrival at the scene, you find a 36-year-old woman in labor. She tells you this is her third pregnancy and that the baby is "on the way."

a. What questions should you ask the mother when deciding whether to transport or assist in delivery on the scene?

_____

_____

_____

b. You prepare for delivery on the scene and advise medical direction. Within a few minutes, the infant's head is being delivered. You find the umbilical cord is wrapped around the infant's neck. What should you do?

_____

_____

_____

c. What are the last steps in the delivery process?

_____

_____

_____

35. You are assisting in the delivery of a multiple birth. The first infant has been delivered, and the baby and mother are doing fine. As the second infant delivers, you note that the color of the infant's neck and trunk is blue and dusky. The baby is not crying, and the mother senses that something is wrong. You suction the mouth and nose, dry the infant, and stimulate breathing. Spontaneous respirations remain inadequate.

a. What is your next step in resuscitation?

_____

_____

b. After a few ventilations the infant begins to cry. What is your next assessment?

_____

_____

c. The baby's color improves, and the baby is beginning to respond appropriately. What is your next step in managing this infant?

_____

_____

DIVISION FOUR EXAMINATION
MEDICAL/BEHAVIORAL
EMERGENCIES AND OBSTETRICS
AND GYNECOLOGY

Directions: Circle the letter of the correct answer.

1. Which of the following medications is carried on the EMS unit?
   a. Nitroglycerin
   b. Activated charcoal
   c. Epinephrine autoinjectors
   d. Inhalers

2. What name of a medication is listed in the *U.S. Pharmacopeia*?
   a. Chemical name
   b. Generic name
   c. Trade name
   d. Brand name

3. A(n) _____ is a situation in which a medication should not be used because it may cause harm to the patient or offer no effect in improving the patient's condition or illness.
   a. Indication
   b. Contraindication
   c. Complication
   d. Association

4. What form of medication is activated charcoal?
   a. Tablet
   b. Gel
   c. Suspension
   d. Sublingual spray

5. Oral medications:
   a. Are sprayed under the tongue
   b. Are useful for unresponsive patients
   c. Have a slow onset of action
   d. Should not be given to alert children

6. Which of the following is true?
   a. Knowing the side effects of a drug will help the EMT–Basic anticipate the onset of these side effects
   b. Side effects are the helpful effects of a drug
   c. The mechanism of action of a drug describes how the drug is eliminated from the body
   d. EMT–Basics can help a patient take any medication if the patient is in acute distress

7. The larynx is also known as the:
   a. Oropharynx
   b. Diaphragm
   c. Windpipe
   d. Voice box

8. Which of the following is true?
   a. Stridor is the noise heard when there is liquid in the back of the throat
   b. Agonal respirations are normal in pediatric patients
   c. A barrel chest may indicate long-term respiratory problems
   d. Do not apply high-flow oxygen to a patient who normally receives low concentration oxygen

9. Which of the following is a sign or symptom associated with adequate breathing?
   a. Shortness of breath for a 44-year-old patient
   b. Increased pulse rate for a 65-year-old patient
   c. Retractions in a 10-year-old patient
   d. Rate of 15 breaths per minute for an 18-year-old patient

10. Medication names such as Proventil and Ventolin are examples of _____ names.
    a. Generic   c. Official
    b. Trade   d. Chemical
11. Which of the following is an indication for assisting a patient with a prescribed inhaler?
    a. The patient is unresponsive and cannot use the device without assistance
    b. Medical direction orders the EMT–Basics to administer an inhaler carried on the EMS unit
    c. The patient has signs and symptoms of a respiratory emergency
    d. The patient has not yet been diagnosed with a respiratory problem requiring an inhaler
12. Common side effects of prescribed inhalers include:
    a. Hypotension   c. Increased pulse rate
    b. Cyanosis   d. Memory disturbances
13. The right ventricle pumps blood to:
    a. The body   c. The right atrium
    b. The lungs   d. The aorta
14. Signs and symptoms of shock (hypoperfusion) include:
    a. Slow, full pulse   c. High temperature
    b. Bright red skin   d. Rapid, shallow breathing
15. How should a patient with a cardiac history be positioned for transport?
    a. Sitting   c. 30° upright
    b. Lying down   d. In a position of comfort
16. Which of the following is an indication or a condition that must be met before assisting a patient with administration of nitroglycerin?
    a. The patient has no chest pain now but had chest pain earlier today
    b. The patient has his/her own physician-prescribed sublingual tablets
    c. The patient has taken the maximum dose with no relief
    d. The patient's blood pressure is 94/60
17. An AED can be used for which of the following patients?
    a. An 80-year-old, 100-lb woman with no pulse
    b. A 50-year-old, 220-lb man who complains of chest pain
    c. A 10-year-old, 36-kg unresponsive patient struck by lightning
    d. A 90-year-old, 75-kg unresponsive man with a pulse
18. How long should the EMT–Basic perform CPR after the first three shocks are delivered?
    a. 30 seconds   c. 90 seconds
    b. 60 seconds   d. 120 seconds
19. Signs and symptoms of a diabetic emergency include:
    a. Lack of appetite   c. Normal heart rate
    b. Intoxicated appearance   d. Hot, dry skin
20. Which of the following medications in a patient's home would alert you that the patient has a history of diabetes?
    a. Ventolin   c. Dilantin
    b. Humulin   d. Procardia
21. Which of the following is a common cause of seizures?
    a. Hypothermia
    b. Infections
    c. Near drowning
    d. Decreased levels of carbon dioxide
22. Which of the following is an indication for the administration of oral glucose?
    a. Patient with a history of diabetes who is unresponsive
    b. Patient with signs and symptoms of hypoglycemia who is unable to swallow
    c. Patient with an altered mental status and a history of diabetes
    d. Patient has an altered mental status with no past medical history

23. What dose of glucose should be given to a patient who is unresponsive?
    a. One tube, placed between the patient's cheek and gum
    b. Two tubes, under the tongue
    c. One tube, under the tongue
    d. Oral glucose is not indicated
24. Which of the following best defines an allergic reaction?
    a. Coughing with dry mucous membranes
    b. A rash on the extremities
    c. Swelling of the face and throat
    d. Exaggerated immune response to any substance
25. When do you assess the SAMPLE history for a patient with an allergic reaction?
    a. During the initial assessment
    b. During the focused history and physical examination
    c. During the detailed physical examination
    d. During the ongoing assessment
26. What dose of epinephrine is found in an adult epinephrine autoinjector?
    a. 0.15 mg   c. 5 mg
    b. 0.3 mg   d. 10 mg
27. Where is the tip of the autoinjector placed on the patient?
    a. Lateral arm   c. Lateral thigh
    b. Lateral buttock   d. Anterior thigh
28. What should be done with the autoinjector after use?
    a. Retract the needle into the injector
    b. Keep with the patient until you reach the hospital
    c. Place in biohazard container
    d. Dispose of the needle separate from the injector
29. Which of the following is a side effect of epinephrine?
    a. Increased heart rate   c. Warm, dry skin
    b. Red, itchy skin   d. Difficulty breathing
30. Which of the following should be determined while caring for a poisoning/overdose patient?
    a. If the poisoning was intentional or accidental
    b. If the parents were negligent, if the patient is a child
    c. How much substance was ingested
    d. Whose medication was taken
31. If the patient exhibits signs and symptoms including diarrhea, abdominal pain, chemical burns around the mouth, and unusual breath odors, which route of poisoning would you suspect?
    a. Inhaled   c. Injected
    b. Ingested   d. Absorbed
32. Which of the following routes for poisoning is an indication for activated charcoal?
    a. Inhaled   c. Absorbed
    b. Injection   d. Ingested
33. What is the dose of activated charcoal for children?
    a. 0.5 g/kg   c. 2 g/kg
    b. 1 g/kg   d. 5 g/kg
34. Which of the following is a common side effect of activated charcoal?
    a. Elevated heart rate   c. Cyanosis around the mouth
    b. Vomiting   d. Unresponsiveness
35. Which of the following is a method of heat loss?
    a. Shivering   c. Conduction
    b. Condensation   d. Conversion

36. Where should the EMT–Basic feel the patient's skin to determine signs and symptoms of generalized hypothermia?
    a. Forehead
    c. Abdomen
    b. Upper arm
    d. Lower leg
37. What are the early signs and symptoms associated with generalized hypothermia?
    a. Rapid pulse, rapid breathing, and red skin
    b. Slow pulse, rapid breathing, and pale skin
    c. Rapid pulse, slow breathing, and cyanotic skin
    d. Slow pulse, slow breathing, and red skin
38. Which of the following is the most serious sign or symptom of generalized hyperthermia?
    a. Muscular cramps
    c. Hot, dry skin
    b. Rapid heart rate
    d. Abdominal cramps
39. Which of the following is true?
    a. The term "drowning" indicates that a patient has lived after an immersion incident
    b. The incidence of spinal injuries is high in water-related emergencies
    c. Gastric distention should be relieved as soon as possible for near-drowning patients
    d. Immersion in warm water will make resuscitation more likely
40. How should you care for an extremity that has a stinger in place from an insect?
    a. Leave it in
    b. Use tweezers to remove it
    c. Use the edge of a card to remove it
    d. Rub it off with your finger
41. Patients considered to be at risk for suicide include:
    a. Patients who are 30 years of age and single
    b. Teenagers
    c. Patients who have had a serious illness for many years
    d. Patients who have lost their jobs
42. Which of the following is a method for calming a patient with a behavioral emergency?
    a. Tell the patient what you are doing
    b. Move close to the patient quickly to gain the patient's trust
    c. Do not answer questions that may upset the patient
    d. Separate the patient from family members or friends
43. Which of the following is true?
    a. Do not assess behavioral emergency patients for injury or illness
    b. Do not question the patient about past medical history because this may upset the patient
    c. Do not use metal handcuffs as restraints
    d. Do not use same-gender attendants for behavioral emergency patients
44. How much force should be used to restrain a patient?
    a. Minimal force
    c. Reasonable force
    b. Maximum force
    d. Force should not be used
45. What is the name of the organ in which the fetus grows and matures?
    a. Amniotic sac
    c. Birth canal
    b. Uterus
    d. Perineum
46. Which of the following is true?
    a. The first stage of labor begins with regular contractions of the uterus
    b. The second stage of labor ends when the baby enters the birth canal
    .c. The third stage of labor begins with the delivery of the placenta
    d. The second stage of labor ends when the cervix is fully dilated

47. Which of the following is **NOT** usually found in an obstetrical kit?
    a. Cord clamps/hemostats   c. Magill forceps
    b. Bulb syringe   d. Baby blanket
48. Which of the following is a consideration for normal delivery?
    a. Prepare the patient for transport if the contractions are less than 2 minutes apart
    b. Do not let the mother go to the bathroom
    c. Do not let the mother push until you arrive at the hospital
    d. If crowning is present, prepare for transport immediately
49. How far from the infant should the cord be cut after delivery?
    a. 2 finger widths
    b. 4 finger widths
    c. Equal distances between mother and infant
    d. Very close to the mother
50. If the mother loses 750 cc of blood during the delivery and she is still bleeding, how should the EMT–Basic manage this patient?
    a. No special management is required, it is normal to lose up to 1000 cc of blood during childbirth
    b. Place gauze into the vaginal opening, and replace the gauze when it becomes soaked with blood
    c. Massage the uterus in a kneading motion
    d. Massage the perineum until the bleeding stops
51. What is the name of the condition when the cord presents through the birth canal before delivery of the head?
    a. Breech cord   c. Cord delivery
    b. Prolapsed cord   d. Meconium birth

DIVISION FIVE
TRAUMA

CHAPTER 25
BLEEDING AND SHOCK

● **CHAPTER OUTLINE**

● MATCHING

Match the terms in Column 1 with the correct definition in Column 2:

Column 1	Column 2
1. _____ Capillary refill	**a.** measure of the perfusion of the skin in a child under 6 years of age
2. _____ Circumferential pressure	**b.** hypoperfusion
3. _____ Epistaxis	**c.** state that results when cells are not receiving adequate blood flow
4. _____ Hemorrhagic shock	**d.** hypoperfusion that results from an inadequate volume of blood
5. _____ Hypoperfusion	**e.** bleeding from the nose
6. _____ Hypovolemic shock	**f.** place in an extremity where a major artery lies close to a bone
7. _____ Perfusion	**g.** pressure around an extremity
8. _____ Pressure point	**h.** hypoperfusion that results from bleeding
9. _____ Shock	**i.** process of delivering oxygen and nutrients to, and removing metabolic waste products from, the body's cells

● REVIEW QUESTIONS

1. The cardiovascular system delivers _____ through a

   system of _____, _____, and capillaries.

2. The average adult has approximately _____ L of blood in the body.
   - **a.** 12
   - **b.** 5
   - **c.** 6
   - **d.** 7

3. The body delivers an equal amount of blood to all parts of the body. **True or false?**

4. The _____ pressure is measured during contraction of the heart, the _____ pressure is measured during the heart's resting phase.
   - **a.** Systolic; diastolic
   - **b.** Diastolic; systolic
   - **c.** Systolic; resting
   - **d.** Beating; diastolic

5. Good perfusion of the body requires an adequate _____.

6. A decrease in perfusion to the cells in the body results in hypoperfusion or

   _____.

7. When tissues are not adequately perfused they are damaged by lack of

   _____ and a build-up of _____

   _____.

8. The four major organs easily damaged by hypoperfusion are:

   a. _____

   b. _____

   c. _____

   d. _____
9. List three causes of hypovolemic shock:

   a. _____

   b. _____

   c. _____
10. Early, subtle signs of shock are anxiety and _____.
    a. Anger   c. Sleepiness
    b. Restlessness   d. Anxiety
11. Vasoconstriction causes blood vessels in the extremities to dilate, producing warm skin. **True or false?**
12. Reduced blood flow to arms and legs results in weaker peripheral pulses compared with central pulses. **True or false?**
13. When assessing the capillary refill of a child, the color will return in _____ for a patient with adequate perfusion.
    a. Less than 2 seconds   c. Less than 4 seconds
    b. Less than 3 seconds   d. Less than 5 seconds
14. Another early sign of shock is an increased _____.
    a. Blood pressure   c. Heart rate
    b. Temperature   d. Mental status

15. A late sign of shock is a _____ blood pressure.

16. The first priority with any patient is to ensure an _____

    _____.

17. The legs can be elevated only if the patient has no serious injuries to the _____. (mark all that apply)
    a. Spine   e. Head
    b. Upper extremities   f. Chest
    c. Pelvis   g. Abdomen
    d. Lower extremities
18. Body substance isolation precautions are very important when caring for a patient with external injuries. **True or false?**

19. For an adult, a sudden loss of _____ L of blood is serious.
20. When bleeding is from an artery the blood will _____.
    a. Drip   c. Spurt
    b. Ooze   d. Flow
21. Venous bleeding will usually _____.
    a. Drip   c. Spurt
    b. Ooze   d. Flow

22. Bleeding that involves the capillaries will usually _____.

23. The most effective method of controlling bleeding from one main artery or major vein is with _____.
    a. Diffuse direct pressure   **c.** Pressure points
    b. Concentrated direct pressure   **d.** Extremity elevation
24. List three ways bleeding from multiple sites on an extremity can be controlled:

    a. _____

    b. _____

    c. _____

25. If there is no pain, swelling, or deformity, _____ can decrease blood flow to an injury.
26. Which type of bleeding control will slow bleeding but rarely stop it completely?
    a. Diffuse direct pressure   **c.** Pressure points
    b. Concentrated direct pressure   **d.** Extremity elevation
27. Splinting an extremity injury stabilizes bone ends and reduces potential for further damage to blood vessels and nerves. **True or false?**
28. An injury to the chest is a contraindication for use of the pneumatic anti-shock garment (PASG). **True or false?**

29. The last resort for bleeding control is a _____.
30. Which of the following is **NOT** a principle of tourniquet use:
    a. It must apply enough continuous circumferential pressure to stop the bleeding
    b. It should be removed once the bleeding has been stopped for 10 minutes
    c. It should be used only after all other measures have failed
    d. Never cover the tourniquet with dressings or blankets

31. If a tourniquet is used, always avoid placing it over a _____ injury.

32. Bleeding from the ears and nose can be a sign of a _____

    _____ in a trauma patient.
33. Direct pressure should be applied to bleeding from the nose and ears. **True or false?**
34. If a patient has signs and symptoms of shock (hypoperfusion) and a serious mechanism of injury, with no obvious bleeding, you should suspect

    _____ _____.
35. List six signs and symptoms of internal bleeding:

    a. _____

    b. _____

    c. _____

    d. _____

    e. _____

    f. _____

36. If you suspect a patient is bleeding internally from an injured femur, how would you treat this patient?

_____

_____

37. When should the PASG be applied?

_____

_____

38. You and your crew have been dispatched to an automobile-pedestrian collision. On arrival, you find an elderly man lying in the roadway at a busy intersection. Police are directing traffic, and the scene is safe. According to witnesses, the patient was struck head-on by a vehicle traveling 10 to 20 miles per hour. There is profuse bleeding from the patient's lower extremities and an obvious open injury to his left thigh with visible bone ends protruding. Due to the patient's age, his apparent blood loss, and the mechanism of injury, you suspect the patient may soon have hypoperfusion.

   a. Airway control and spinal immobilization are your first priorities in caring for this patient. What role does providing oxygen play in managing shock?

_____

_____

   b. You attempt to control bleeding by applying diffuse direct pressure to the patient's wounds. The bleeding, however, continues. What will be your next step in providing hemorrhage control?

_____

_____

   c. It is obvious that the patient needs rapid transport for definitive care. Medical direction advises you to apply and inflate the pneumatic anti-shock garment (PASG). How will the PASG benefit this patient?

_____

_____

39. You are caring for an elderly patient who has had bloody stools for the past 12 hours. She is pale, diaphoretic, and extremely weak. She describes the bloody stools as "bright-red diarrhea." She has no past significant medical history and denies any pain. Her vital signs are blood pressure 106/70, pulse 120, and respirations 22 and shallow.

   a. Based on the patient's description of her bleeding, where do you suspect to be the source of her bleeding?

_____

_____

_____

b. What is the significance of the patient's vital signs?

_____

_____

c. How would you manage this patient?

_____

_____

CHAPTER 26

SOFT-TISSUE INJURIES

● **CHAPTER OUTLINE**

I. The Skin

    A. Function

    B. Layers

II. Injuries

    A. Closed Injuries

        1. Contusion

        2. Hematoma

        3. Closed crush injury

    B. Open Injuries

        1. Abrasion

        2. Laceration

        3. Avulsion

        4. Penetration or puncture

        5. Amputation

        6. Open crush injury

    C. Emergency Medical Care for Patients With Soft-Tissue Injuries

        1. Dressings and bandages

        2. Injuries requiring special consideration

III. Burns

    A. Classification of Burns

    B. Severity of Burns

        1. Critical burns

        2. Moderate burns

        3. Minor burns

    C. Emergency Medical Care for Burn Victims

● MATCHING

Match the terms in Column 1 with the correct definition in Column 2:

Column 1	Column 2
1. _____ Abrasion	**a.** open soft-tissue injury resulting from a scraping force
2. _____ Amputation	**b.** sterile material used to control bleeding and protect soft-tissue injury
3. _____ Avulsion	**c.** open or closed soft-tissue injury resulting from blunt force trauma
4. _____ Bandage	**d.** flap of skin that is torn or pulled loose
5. _____ Contusion	**e.** open wound in the abdomen through which organs are protruding
6. _____ Crush injury	**f.** material used to secure a dressing in place
7. _____ Dressing	**g.** burn that affects only the epidermis
8. _____ Evisceration	**h.** break in the skin of varying depth caused by a sharp object; a cut
9. _____ Full-thickness burn	**i.** burn that affects all layers of the skin
10. _____ Hematoma	**j.** removal of an appendage from the body
11. _____ Laceration	**k.** open soft-tissue injury caused by an object being pushed into skin
12. _____ Occlusive	**l.** burn that affects the epidermis and dermis
13. _____ Partial-thickness burn	**m.** type of closed soft-tissue injury; a bruise
14. _____ Penetration or puncture	**n.** referring to protection from the air
15. _____ Superficial burn	**o.** closed soft-tissue injury where large blood vessels are injured, with 1 L or more of blood under the skin

● REVIEW QUESTIONS

1. List three functions of the skin:

   a. _____

   b. _____

   c. _____

2. Nerve endings can be found in which layer of the skin?
   a. Epidermis
   b. Dermis
   c. Subcutaneous
   d. There are no nerve endings in the skin

3. Define a closed injury:

   _____

4. A discoloration to the skin with minimal pain and swelling is called a(n):
   a. Contusion　　c. Crush injury
   b. Hematoma　　d. Abrasion

5. A large collection of blood under the skin, up to 1 L, is called a(n):
   a. Contusion   c. Crush injury
   b. Hematoma   d. Abrasion
6. Define an open injury:

   _____

7. The scraping wound caused by falling on asphalt is a(n) _____.
   a. Penetration/puncture   c. Crush injury
   b. Abrasion   d. Amputation
8. The type of wound commonly called a "cut" is a(n):
   a. Avulsion   c. Laceration
   b. Abrasion   d. Amputation
9. A gunshot wound is an example of a(n):
   a. Penetration/puncture   c. Crush injury
   b. Abrasion   d. Amputation
10. The loss of a finger is called a(n):
    a. Penetration/puncture   c. Laceration
    b. Abrasion   d. Amputation
11. Body substance isolation precautions are a necessary part of preparing to care for a soft-tissue injury. **True or false?**
12. An appropriately sized dressing should just barely cover the wound. **True or false?**
13. List three ways to apply a pressure dressing:

    a. _____

    b. _____

    c. _____

14. An occlusive dressing, taped on _____ sides, allows

    air to _____ but not _____
    the wound.
15. Protect eviscerated organs with a dry, sterile dressing. **True or false?**
16. List two of the conditions under which an impaled object should be removed:

    a. _____

    b. _____
17. For an impaled object in the eye, the uninjured eye is also covered to:
    a. Keep the patient quiet
    b. Reduce movement of both eyes
    c. Keep the patient from seeing the injury
    d. Reduce sensory stimulus
18. Amputated parts should be placed in cold water for transport. **True or false?**
19. When caring for a patient with an evisceration, chest injury, or burn, the pri-

    ority for care is always to maintain the patient's _____.
20. Partial amputations should be _____ and _____.
    a. Splinted; completed   c. Completed; bandaged
    b. Immobilized; bandaged   d. None of the above
21. Direct pressure can be used on the head only if there is no evidence of a

    _____.

22. Injuries to the mouth should be evaluated for _____ and _____.
    a. Bleeding; foreign objects
    c. Dentures; impaled objects
    b. Loose teeth; bleeding
    d. Foreign objects; airway obstruction
23. List five criteria used to determine the severity of a burn:

    a. _____

    b. _____

    c. _____

    d. _____

    e. _____

24. A sunburn is a type of _____ burn.
25. Dry, leathery, charred skin with little or no pain describes a

    _____ burn.

26. If blisters form, the burn is considered to be a _____
    burn.
27. In the "Rule of Nines" the head of an adult is _____ %

    of the body surface area and the head of an infant is _____%.
28. A circumferential burn of the torso wraps all the way around and could
    cause respiratory difficulty. **True or false?**
29. List five areas of the body that are considered critical if burned:

    a. _____

    b. _____

    c. _____

    d. _____

    e. _____
30. Determine the severity of each burn described below. (c=critical; mod =
    moderate; min = minor)

    _____ A partial-thickness burn of the face

    _____ A child with a partial thickness burn of less than 10%

    _____ A Full-thickness burn of less than 2%

    _____ A Partial-thickness burn covering 27% of the body
31. Because of skin loss with a burn, patients must be protected from _____.
    a. Hypothermia
    c. Shivering
    b. Hyperthermia
    d. None of the above
32. Jewelry and clothing should be removed when treating a burn patient. **True
    or false?**
33. If a patient has suffered a chemical burn from dry powder, first

    _____ the powder, then _____
    with water.

34. When treating a patient with _____ burns, be prepared with the AED because cardiac arrest is a possibility.

35. You are caring for a worker who has fallen from a mowing tractor. As he fell, his right foot was caught in the machine producing a large open wound to his foot and ankle. The bones of his ankle and lower extremity are exposed, and the wound is full of grass and debris. He is in extreme pain and says that he cannot feel or move his toes. You begin to remove his shoe when you realize that his foot is nearly amputated.

    a. Describe general principles of emergency care for patients with soft-tissue injury.

_____

_____

    b. You attempt to control his bleeding with direct pressure, but the dressing continues to become saturated with blood. What should you do?

_____

_____

    c. The patient is starting to look a little "shocky." What should you do?

_____

_____

36. You are caring for a firefighter who was trapped in a burning building. She has partial- and full-thickness burns over her anterior chest and abdomen, right arm, and leg.

    a. Define partial-thickness and full-thickness burns.

_____

_____

    b. Using the "Rule of Nines," what percentage of body area is burned?

_____

_____

    c. Describe emergency care for burn patients.

_____

_____

MUSCULOSKELETAL CARE

● **CHAPTER OUTLINE**

I. Musculoskeletal Review

    A. The Muscular System

    B. The Skeletal System

II. Injuries to Bones and Joints

    A. Mechanism of Injury

    B. Bone or Joint Injuries

    C. Emergency Care for Patients With Bone or Joint Injuries

III. Splinting an Injury

    A. Reasons for Splinting

    B. Principles of Splinting

    C. Equipment and Techniques

    D. Risks of Splinting

● MATCHING

Match the terms in Column 1 with the correct definition in Column 2:

Column 1	Column 2
1. _____ Angulation	**a.** injury that results from a force that comes into direct contact with an area of the body
2. _____ Closed injury	**b.** injury in one body area that results from a force that comes into contact with a different part of the body
3. _____ Crepitation	**c.** type of splint that does not conform to the body
4. _____ Direct injury	**d.** injury that breaks the continuity of the skin
5. _____ Indirect injury	**e.** sound made when bone ends rub together or when there is air inside the tissue
6. _____ Mechanism of injury	**f.** force that acts on the body to produce an injury
7. _____ Open injury	**g.** bandaging used to immobilize a shoulder or arm injury
8. _____ Pneumatic splints	**h.** special device used to immobilize a closed midfemur injury
9. _____ Position of function	**i.** injury that does not break the continuity of the skin
10. _____ Rigid splints	**j.** injury that is deformed (bent) at the site
11. _____ Sling and swathe	**k.** devices such as air or vacuum splints that conform to the injury
12. _____ Traction splints	**l.** injury that results from a turning motion of the body in opposite directions
13. _____ Twisting injury	**m.** relaxed position of the hand or foot in which there is minimal movement or stretching of muscle

● REVIEW QUESTIONS

1. List three functions of muscles:

   a. _____

   b. _____

   c. _____

2. Skeletal muscles are attached to _____ and are

   responsible for _____.

3. Muscles that we have no direct control over are called _____,

   or _____, muscles.

4. Automaticity is a characteristic only found in _____
   muscle.

5. Label Figure 27-1 with the following terms:

clavicle	tibia
scapula	fibula
sternum	humerus
vertebral column	radius
femur	ulna
patella	

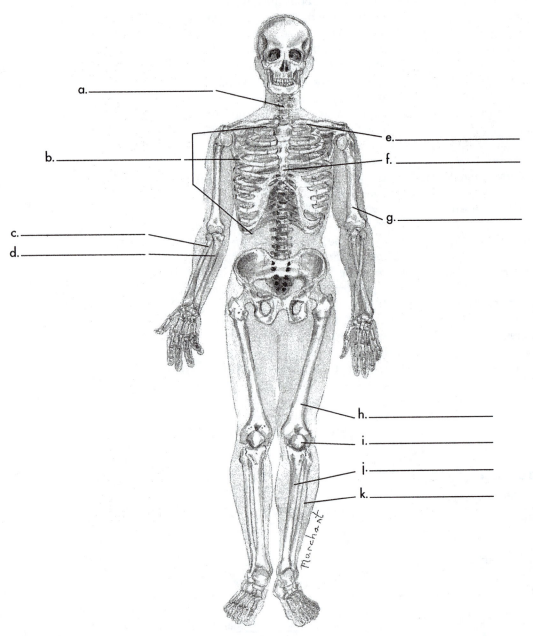

a. _____

b. _____

c. _____

d. _____

e. _____

f. _____

g. _____

h. _____

i. _____

j. _____

k. _____

Figure 27-1 From Sorrentino: *Mosby's Textbook for Nursing Assistants*, 4/e, 1996, Mosby Lifeline.

6. Label Figure 27-2 with the following terms:
   cervical vertebrae   sacral vertebrae
   thoracic vertebrae   fused coccyx
   lumbar vertebrae

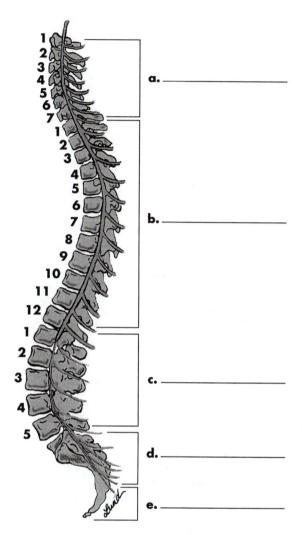

a. _____

b. _____

c. _____

d. _____

e. _____

Figure 27-2

7. List three functions of the skeletal system:

   a. _____

   b. _____

   c. _____

8. The knee is an example of a _____ joint, and the hip

   is a _____ joint.

9. Match the mechanism of injury in column 1 with the correct example in column 2:

Column 1

a. Direct injury
b. Twisting injury
c. Indirect injury

Column 2

_____ fist to the jaw

_____ internal organs against the chest in an automobile crash

_____ running back tackled after turning from a catch

10. List four signs and symptoms of a musculoskeletal injury:

a. _____

b. _____

c. _____

d. _____

11. Splinting painful, swollen extremities should always begin after an evaluation of airway and breathing. **True or false?**

12. Splinting _____ movement of bone fragments and

_____ damage to muscles and nerves.

13. Pulse, motor function, and sensation must be evaluated _____

and _____ splinting.

14. If the distal pulse changes after splinting, _____ the splint and reassess.

15. The position of function for the hand is with the fingers extended. **True or false?**

16. To be effective, a splint must immobilize the joint _____

and _____ a long bone injury.

17. Full body immobilization should be used if _____ trauma is suspected.

18. A traction splint can be used if _____.
    a. The injury is at or near a joint
    b. The injury is closed and near midfemur
    c. The injury also involves the lower leg
    d. The injury is open with exposed bone ends

19. Pneumatic splints are flexible and good for immobilization of

_____ injuries.

20. List at least two advantages of a pneumatic splint:

a. _____

b. _____

21. The pneumatic anti-shock garment (PASG) can be used as an immobilization device. **True or false?**

22. Shoulder injuries usually require a _____ _____

_____for stabilization.

23. List three risks of splints that are too tight, too loose, or improperly applied:

a. _____

b. _____

c. _____

24. You have been dispatched to the local skating rink where a 12-year-old boy has fallen and injured his arm. He tells you that he lost his balance and tried to "catch himself" as he fell backward. His right arm is angulated and swollen and deformed at the wrist. There are no other apparent injuries. He denies hitting his head or losing responsiveness.

a. What are signs and symptoms of a bone or joint injury?

_____

_____

b. What type of assessment is required for this injury?

_____

_____

c. Describe how you would splint this injury.

_____

_____

_____

CHAPTER 28
INJURIES TO THE HEAD AND SPINE

● **CHAPTER OUTLINE**

I. Review of the Nervous and Skeletal Systems

   A. The Nervous System

   B. The Skeletal System

II. Devices for Immobilization

   A. Cervical Spine

   B. Short Backboards

   C. Long Backboards (Full-Body Spinal Immobilization Devices)

III. Injuries to the Spine

   A. Mechanism of Injury

   B. Assessment

      1. Signs and symptoms

      2. Responsive patients

      3. Unresponsive patients

   C. Complications

   D. Emergency Medical Care of the Spine-Injured Patient

IV. Injuries to the Brain and Skull

   A. Head and Skull Injuries

   B. Emergency Medical Care of the Head-Injured Patient

V. Special Considerations

   A. Rapid Extrication

   B. Helmet Removal

   C. Infants and Children

   D. Geriatric Patients

● MATCHING

Match the following terms in Column 1 with the correct definition in Column 2:

	Column 1		Column 2
1. _____	Cervical spine immobilization device	a.	a full-body spinal immobilization device
2. _____	Kendrick Extrication Device (KED)	b.	method used to move a lying patient onto a long board
3. _____	Long backboard	c.	technique used to rapidly move a patient from a scene
4. _____	Log roll	d.	device used to maintain immobilization of the head, neck, and torso
5. _____	Rapid extrication	e.	device used to maintain immobilization of the head and neck
6. _____	Short backboard	f.	type of short board used to immobilize a seated patient

● REVIEW QUESTIONS

1. The components of the central nervous system are _____

   and the _____ _____.

2. Cerebrospinal fluid (CSF) surrounds the _____ and

   spinal cord and acts as a _____.
3. Sensory nerves carry information (to/from) the body (to/from) the brain.

4. The spinal column contains _____ bones.
5. Indicate the number of bones in each section of the vertebral column.

   _____ Cervical   _____ Sacral

   _____ Thoracic   _____ Coccygeal

   _____ Lumbar
6. Cervical spine immobilization devices provide adequate immobilization for the head, and the patient requires no manual stabilization. **True or false?**
7. A short backboard is used to immobilize the head, neck, and torso when the

   patient is in a _____ position.

8. Long backboards provide _____ body immobilization.
9. Adequate immobilization of the spine requires only a cervical spine immobilization device and long backboard. **True or false?**
10. Define mechanism of injury:

_____

11. The mechanism of injury helps you understand _____.
    a. If the patient truly could be hurt
    b. If there was a significant force applied to the body
    c. If you should be concerned about the patient
    d. None of the above

12. List four significant mechanisms of injury:

   a. _____

   b. _____

   c. _____

   d. _____

13. Match the mechanism of injury with the type of incident:

   _____ hanging   **a.** compression

                         b. distraction

   _____ shallow water diving   **c.** excessive flexion, extension

   _____ rear-end automobile crash

14. Never ask a patient to move to determine if he/she has pain in a particular area. **True or false?**

15. Injuries to the shoulder and chest could indicate the possibility of an injury

   to the _____.

16. Numbness, tingling, or weakness are possible signs and symptoms of a

   _____.

17. List five important questions to ask during an assessment of a responsive trauma patient.

   a. _____

   b. _____

   c. _____

   d. _____

   e. _____

18. Define each of the letters in the acronym DCAP-BTLS:

   D _____ B _____

   C _____ T _____

   A _____ L _____

   P _____ S _____

19. After every intervention, assess _____ _____,

   _____ _____, and _____

   _____.

20. You must document all findings and any changes in patient status during care and treatment. **True or false?**

21. It helps to complete the assessment of the cervical region

   _____ (after/prior to) application of the cervical spine immobilization device.

22. Why is it especially important to monitor the respirations of a potentially spine injured patient?

_____

_____

23. Which of the following statements about cervical spine immobilization device is true?
    a. They should be used for patients who may have sustained head, neck, or back injuries
    b. Most do not need to be sized
    c. The patient's head must be straightened to measure for it, even if this causes pain
    d. Manual spinal stabilization can be released once it is in place
24. Which of the following statements about log rolls and spinal immobilization is true?
    a. The EMT–Basic controlling the patient's shoulders is responsible for calling out when to move the patient
    b. If the patient is not on the center of the long backboard after log rolling, move the patient by pushing on the shoulder and hip until the patient is centered
    c. The patient's head should be immobilized to the board after the shoulders and hips
    d. The patient's legs should be immobilized to the board prior to immobilizing the shoulders
25. Number the steps in the immobilization of a patient with a short backboard in order, with 1 as the first step and 7 as the last:

    _____ Secure the torso to the board

    _____ Place the spine board behind the patient

    _____ Reassess pulse, motor function and sensation

    _____ Secure the arms, legs, and feet

    _____ Pad the voids behind the patient's head

    _____ Attach the straps to the board

    _____ Secure the head to the board

26. To immobilize a seated patient you can use a _____

    _____ or a _____ _____.
27. Patients immobilized to short spine boards or vest type devices must be

    secured to a _____ _____
    for transport.

28. Spinal injuries also may involve injuries to the _____

    and _____.
29. Scalp wounds bleed little because there are few blood vessels located in the scalp. **True or false?**
30. The best indicator of a traumatic head injury is _____.

31. List five signs and symptoms of a traumatic head injury:

   a. _____

   b. _____

   c. _____

   d. _____

   e. _____

32. List three situations when rapid extrication should be used:

   a. _____

   b. _____

   c. _____

33. In which of the following situations should a helmet be left in place?
   a. When the patient complains of neck pain
   b. Any time the patient is unresponsive
   c. When removal would cause further injury
   d. When the helmet fits loosely and is comfortable for the patient
34. Which of the following is true regarding helmets and helmet removal?
   a. Sports helmets are typically open in the front, making the airway easy to access
   b. Full face shield helmets typically should be left in place
   c. If the helmet is left in place, a commercial cervical spine immobilization device will provide good immobilization of the helmet to the long backboard
   d. Shoulder pads should be left in place when a football helmet is removed
35. How is the head immobilized while the helmet is being removed?
   a. With one hand on the forehead and one under the jaw
   b. With both hands under the neck
   c. With one hand on the mandible and the other on the occipital region
   d. By placing one hand on either side of the helmet, without touching the face or head
36. For an infant or small child, padding may have to be placed under the

   _____ to _____ to maintain neutral alignment.
37. Neutral alignment in the elderly may be difficult due to changes in the spine from disease. **True or false?**
38. You have been dispatched to the scene of an "injured child." En route, you are advised that a 10-year-old girl has fallen from the back of a moving pickup truck. On arrival, the distraught father is holding the child in his arms. She is unresponsive and has noisy respirations, and there is an obvious open scalp wound with moderate bleeding. With spinal precautions, you and your partner move the child to a spine board and place her in the ambulance.
   a. What is your first priority of care in managing this patient?

_____

_____

b. You suction the child's airway and assist her respirations with a BVM. How would you control the bleeding from her scalp?

_____

_____

c. En route to the emergency department, you continue your assessment and management of this patient. What signs and symptoms of traumatic head injury should you anticipate?

_____

_____

DIVISION FIVE EXAMINATION
TRAUMA

Directions: Circle the letter of the correct answer.

1. Which of the following is true?
   a. All organs need to be equally perfused to function properly
   b. The average adult has about 10 L of blood in the body
   c. Hypovolemic shock occurs when there is not enough blood in the body
   d. The brain, heart, lungs, and kidneys tolerate well an interruption in blood supply
2. Changes in mental status:
   a. Are due to changes in perfusion of the brain
   b. Occur late in shock
   c. Typically occur after a drop in blood pressure
   d. Are a sign of good brain perfusion
3. Signs and symptoms of shock include:
   a. Strong, regular peripheral pulses with weak central pulses
   b. Capillary refill greater than 0.5 seconds in children
   c. Dry skin
   d. Restlessness
4. When treating a patient with signs and symptoms of shock including a low blood pressure:
   a. Position the patient sitting upright to make breathing easier
   b. Provide high-flow oxygen
   c. Keep the patient cool
   d. Splint all extremity injuries on scene to minimize blood loss
5. Which of the following is true?
   a. Blood loss of 1 L is considered serious in adult patients
   b. Geriatric patients tolerate blood loss better than younger patients
   c. Children bleed more slowly than adults
   d. Infants can lose up to 500 mL of blood before it is considered serious
6. This type of bleeding is bright red in color, may spurt with each heart beat, and is difficult to control:
   a. Venous bleeding   c. Capillary bleeding
   b. Arterial bleeding   d. Pulmonary bleeding
7. What is the most effective method to control bleeding from one main source?
   a. Fingertip pressure directly on the point of bleeding
   b. Elevation of the extremity
   c. Pressure points
   d. Tourniquet
8. Which of the following statements about tourniquets is true?
   a. Tourniquets are usually needed in cases of amputation
   b. A piece of rope or wire is an effective tourniquet
   c. Tourniquets cause little tissue damage if left in place less than 10 hours
   d. Areas distal to a tourniquet may need to be amputated
9. Which of the following is true?
   a. Care for epistaxis includes having the patient tilt his/her head back
   b. There can be up to 1 L of blood lost in a closed injury to the tibia
   c. Patients should be treated for hemorrhagic shock only if external bleeding is observed
   d. Vomit that looks like coffee grounds may be a sign of internal bleeding

10. The outer layer of the skin is the:
    a. Epidermis   c. Endodermis
    b. Dermis   d. Subcutaneous
11. A(n) _____ is an injury in which the outermost layers of the skin are scraped away, with little bleeding.
    a. Contusion   c. Abrasion
    b. Crush injury   d. Avulsion
12. Which of the following is an example of a closed injury?
    a. Abrasion   c. Contusion
    b. Laceration   d. Avulsion
13. In this type of injury the skin or tissue is torn loose or pulled completely off:
    a. Laceration   c. Contusion
    b. Amputation   d. Avulsion
14. Which of the following is true?
    a. Dressings are used to secure bandages in place
    b. An occlusive dressing is made of porous material to allow air to pass through
    c. Splint extremity injuries to minimize bleeding
    d. Straighten a joint that is injured before applying bandaging
15. A(n) _____ is an abdominal injury in which the organs are protruding through the wound.
    a. Evisceration   c. Avulsion
    b. Amputation   d. Penetration
16. How should you treat a patient with an impaled object in the cheek?
    a. Leave the impaled object as found
    b. Remove the impaled object
    c. Stabilize the object from inside the mouth
    d. Stabilize the object from outside the mouth
17. How should you care for an amputated finger?
    a. Place the finger in a hot pack to keep it warm
    b. Place the finger in plastic and keep it cool
    c. Place the finger on ice so that it freezes as soon as possible
    d. Place the finger in a bag of ice and water so it will be cool without freezing
18. What type of burn is characterized by intense pain, white to red skin, and blisters?
    a. Superficial burn   c. Full-thickness burn
    b. Partial-thickness burn   d. Full-contact burn
19. You are assessing a 2-month-old patient, who has circumferential burns on both legs and one arm. Using the Rule of Nines, what percentage body surface is burned.
    a. 24%   c. 37%
    b. 30%   d. 43%
20. Which of the following statements about burns is true?
    a. A partial-thickness burn involving the feet is a critical burn
    b. A burn caused by dry lime should be flushed with large amounts of water
    c. Electrical burns cause extensive skin damage but little internal damage
    d. Keep burn patients cool to minimize pain
21. Involuntary muscles:
    a. Are attached to bones to provide movement
    b. Have automaticity and cause the heart to beat
    c. Carry out automatic muscular functions of the body
    d. Are also known as skeletal muscle

22. Which of the following is an example of a direct injury?
    a. Injury to the knee caused by striking the dashboard
    b. Injury to the pelvis caused by the knees striking the dashboard
    c. Injury to an arm caused by pulling and twisting
    d. Injury to the spine caused when landing on the feet from a fall
23. Crepitation is:
    a. Sound heard when there is water under an injury
    b. Sound of bone ends rubbing together
    c. Sound of fluid in the lungs
    d. Sound made when there is swelling in the airway
24. Which of the following statements about splinting is true?
    a. Assess proximal pulse, sensation, and motor function before and after splinting
    b. Splint the bone above and below a joint injury
    c. Replace protruding bone ends before splinting
    d. Leave clothing in place to minimize pain when splinting
25. What should be done for a patient who has multiple extremity injuries and signs and symptoms of shock?
    a. Splint each extremity before transport
    b. Splint the extremities to the long backboard
    c. Splint the upper extremities before transport
    d. Splint the lower extremities before transport
26. For which of the following injuries would you use a traction splint?
    a. Closed injury of the midthigh   c. Injury to lower leg
    b. Injury to thigh and knee   d. Injury to hip
27. The central nervous system is composed of:
    a. Brain and spinal cord
    b. Brain and peripheral nerves
    c. Spinal cord and sensory nerves
    d. Sensory and motor nerves
28. A properly sized cervical spine immobilization device:
    a. Allows the chin to move in and out of the chin rest
    b. Restricts the patient's side-to-side head motion only
    c. Will immobilize the patient's head in a neutral position
    d. Will provide complete immobilization of the head
29. What should be done for the patient if you do not have the proper size cervical spine immobilization devixe?
    a. Instruct the patient not to move his/her head
    b. Use a towel roll and tape
    c. Use a device that is one size too large
    d. Use a device that is one size too small
30. Which of the following statements about short and long backboards is true?
    a. Secure the patient's head to the short board, then secure the body
    b. When using a long backboard, it is not necessary to use a cervical spine immobilization device
    c. When using a KED, buckle the top chest strap before the other chest straps
    d. Reassess distal pulses after immobilizing a patient with a long backboard
31. If a patient hit his/her head on the bottom of a pool while diving, the mechanism of injury to the spine would be:
    a. Extension   c. Distraction
    b. Compression   d. Flexion

32. Which of the following is true?
    a. Patients with no neck or back pain most likely do not have spinal cord damage
    b. Begin manual stabilization of the head after completing the initial assessment
    c. Reassess pulse, motor function, and sensation after every intervention
    d. If the patient's injury is to the pelvis, spinal trauma can be ruled out
33. Use rapid extrication when:
    a. The scene is unsafe for the EMT–Basic to enter
    b. The patient complains of pain in the neck or back
    c. You cannot care for the patient in the position he/she is in
    d. The patient has a head injury
34. Which of the following statements about helmet removal is true?
    a. Football helmets should always be removed
    b. Remove the helmet if it restricts head movement
    c. Helmets should only be removed by athletic trainers
    d. Helmets are removed if the head cannot be immobilized
35. Which of the following is true?
    a. When immobilizing children, pad under the head to achieve a neutral position
    b. Attempt to straighten the spine of geriatric patients for good immobilization
    c. Leave the straps loose when immobilizing children so they do not fight
    d. Children have larger heads in proportion to their body, requiring special immobilization techniques

DIVISION SIX
INFANTS AND CHILDREN

CHAPTER 29
INFANT AND CHILD EMERGENCY CARE

● **CHAPTER OUTLINE**

I. Developmental Differences in Infants and Children

   A. Newborns and Infants

   B. Toddlers

   C. Preschool Children

   D. School-Age Children

   E. Adolescents

II. The Airway

   A. Anatomic and Physiological Concerns

   B. Opening the Airway

   C. Suctioning

   D. Using Airway Adjuncts

      1. Oropharyngeal airway

      2. Nasopharyngeal airway

III. Oxygen Therapy

   A. Blow-by Oxygen

   B. Nonrebreather Masks

   C. Artificial Ventilations

IV. Assessment

V. Common Problems in Infants and Children

   A. Airway Obstruction

      1. Partial obstruction

      2. Complete obstruction

   B. Respiratory Emergencies

      1. Assessment of respiratory problems

      2. Emergency care for patients with respiratory problems

C. Seizures

D. Altered Mental Status

E. Poisoning

F. Fever

G. Shock

H. Near Drowning

I. Sudden Infant Death Syndrome

VI. Trauma

    A. Head Injury

        1. Emergency care for patients with head injury

    B. Chest Injury

        1. Emergency care for patients with chest injury

    C. Abdominal Injury

    D. Burns

        1. Emergency care for burn victims

    E. Other Trauma Considerations

VII. Child Abuse and Neglect

    A. Signs and Symptoms of Child Abuse and Neglect

    B. Emergency Care for Abused and Neglected Patients

VIII. Infants and Children With Special Needs

    A. Tracheostomy Tube

    B. Home Mechanical Ventilators

    C. Central Lines

    D. Gastrostomy Tubes and Gastric Feeding

    E. Shunts

IX. Reactions to Ill and Injured Infants and Children

A. The Family's Reaction

B. The Emergency Medical Technician's Reaction

● MATCHING

Match the terms in Column 1 with the correct definition in Column 2:

Column 1

1. _____ Adolescent

2. _____ Blow-by oxygen

3. _____ Central lines

4. _____ Child abuse

5. _____ Drowning

6. _____ Gastric tube

7. _____ Grunting

8. _____ Infant

9. _____ Nasal flaring

10. _____ Near drowning

11. _____ Neglect

12. _____ Newborn

13. _____ Preschool child

14. _____ Respiratory failure

15. _____ Respiratory distress

16. _____ Retractions

17. _____ School-age child

18. _____ Secondary drowning

19. _____ Shunt

20. _____ Sudden Infant Death Syndrome

21. _____ Toddler

Column 2

a. child 12 to 18 years of age

b. survival past 24 hours after suffocation due to submersion

c. clinical condition in which the infant or child begins to increase the work of breathing

d. used for feeding, way to place food directly into the stomach

e. tube running from the brain to the abdomen to drain excess cerebrospinal fluid

f. child from 6 to 12 years of age

g. sound made when patient in respiratory distress attempts to trap air to keep alveoli open

h. use of accessory muscles to increase the work of breathing

i. attempt by the infant to increase the size of the airway by expanding the nostrils

j. improper or excessive action by parents, guardians, or caretakers that injures or causes harm to children

k. act of not giving attention to a child's essential needs

l. rapid deterioration of respiratory status from several hours to 96 hours after resuscitation

m. term for an infant from birth to 1 month of age

n. method of oxygen delivery for infants and children without placing a mask on the face

o. death from suffocation within the first 24 hours of submersion in liquid

p. sudden, unexplained death of an infant with no discernable cause

q. child from 3 to 6 years of age

r. Intravenous lines surgically placed near the heart for long-term use

s. child less than 1 year of age

t. child 1 to 3 years of age

u. clinical condition when the patient is continuing to work hard to breathe, the effort of breathing is increased, and the patient's condition begins to deteriorate

● REVIEW QUESTIONS

1. Infants must be assessed and treated in a manner to avoid hypothermia. **True or false?**

2. To get the most information about an infant or newborn, assess the

   _____ and _____ first and

   move to the _____ last.

3. List three way to evaluate a child's respirations without touching the patient:

   a. _____

   b. _____

   c. _____

4. Most toddlers do not mind being touched by strangers. **True or false?**

5. The parent can be the most help in the evaluation of a toddler. **True or false?**

6. Most preschoolers like to _____ and will often be

   easily _____ by your equipment.

7. Unlike toddlers and preschoolers, school-age children will be able to relate a good history about what happened. **True or false?**

8. Match the developmental age of the child to the child's need for parents:

   _____ School-age   a. will not be separated from parents
                            b. wants to be separated from parents
   _____ Adolescent   c. will be okay without parents, wants them
                               there
   _____ Infant   d. better in parent's arms

   _____ Toddler

9. The most important differences between infants and children and adults

   involve the _____.

10. Compared with an adult, the airway of a child is _____ and _____ blocked by secretions and swelling.
    a. Larger; more easily   c. Larger; not easily
    b. Smaller; more easily   d. Smaller; not easily

11. In infants and children, the _____ are relatively _____ in relation to the mouth as compared with adults.
    a. Teeth; large   c. Gums; small
    b. Mouth; large   d. Tongue; large

12. In children, drowsiness and tolerance with examination procedures can be a

    sign of _____.

13. To prevent occlusion or kinking of the airway, a head-tilt, chin-lift maneuver

    should put the head into a _____ position, in which
    the nose points straight up.

14. Whenever you suction an infant or child, measure the catheter prior to insertion and suction only as far as you can see. **True or false?**

15. Suctioning should be limited to _____ seconds, and

    you should always apply _____ before and after.

16. To insert an oropharyngeal airway in an infant or child, first (depress/lift) the tongue and insert the airway (with/without) rotation.

17. Nasopharyngeal airways can be used when the patient has a

_____ _____, but oropharyngeal airways cannot.

18. Blow-by oxygen allows delivery of oxygen to an infant or child without placing a mask directly on the child's face. **True or false?**

19. For infants, the rate of flow for blow-by oxygen should be _____ L/min and _____ L/min for children.
    - **a.** 5; 8
    - **c.** 4; 8
    - **b.** 5; 10
    - **d.** 6; 12

20. The recommended rate for artificial ventilation in infants and children is once every _____ seconds or _____ times a minute.
    - **a.** 3; 12
    - **c.** 2; 28
    - **b.** 3; 20
    - **d.** 4; 15

21. Besides the gentle rise of the chest, other indicators of adequate ventilation

in children are improvement in the _____

_____ and _____ _____.

22. With children, consider examining painful areas _____.

23. Define the following letters associated with the mental status acronym:

A _____

V _____

P _____

U _____

24. Indicate if the patients described below have a partial (P) upper airway obstruction; complete (C) upper airway obstruction; or lower (L) airway obstruction:

_____ Stridor on inspiration

_____ Expiratory wheeze

_____ Unable to cough or speak

_____ Skin may appear normal or cyanotic

_____ Skin may appear pale or cyanotic

25. Which of the following statements concerning foreign body airway obstruction is true?
    - **a.** Unresponsive infants should receive back blows and abdominal thrusts for complete airway obstruction
    - **b.** Use abdominal thrusts for a responsive child with an obstruction as you would for an adult
    - **c.** Blind finger sweeps should be performed for infants when there is a known history of foreign body obstruction
    - **d.** When performing abdominal thrusts on the unresponsive child, use the heel of two hands and give 6 to 10 thrusts before inspecting the airway

26. More than 80% of all cardiac arrests in children begin as _____ arrests.

27. List four signs of early respiratory distress in children:

   a. _____

   b. _____

   c. _____

   d _____

28. List four signs of respiratory failure in children:

   a. _____

   b. _____

   c. _____

   d _____

29. A seizure can be caused by a rapid rise in a _____.

30. Which of the following statements is true concerning seizures in pediatric patients:
   a. Always place patients in the recovery position following seizures because there is rarely associated trauma
   b. A bite block inserted into the patient's mouth can be helpful in controlling the airway
   c. A nasopharyngeal airway can be helpful in keeping the tongue off of the back of the throat following a seizure
   d. Seizures are rarely dangerous, even if they last for 30 minutes of more

31. List three common signs and symptoms of shock in an infant or child:

   a. _____

   b. _____

   c. _____

32. The top priority in the treatment of near-drowning cases is adequate

   _____ and _____.

33. Sudden infant death syndrome (SIDS) usually occurs in patients less than _____ months of age.
   a. 12   c. 20
   b. 18   d. 24

34. Because it is larger and heavier than the other parts of the body, the

   _____ is the most frequently injured part of a child's body.

35. When a child has been burned, the biggest concern after airway and breathing is _____.
   a. Hyperthermia   c. Hypothermia
   b. Hypovolemia   d. Vomiting

36. List an indication for use of the PASG in a child:

37. List three signs of child abuse:

    a. _____

    b. _____

    c. _____

38. Most parents feel a sense of loss of control and helplessness when their child is sick or injured. **True or false?**

39. You have been dispatched to a "child with seizures." On arrival, the listless child is being held by a grandparent. The grandmother tells you that the 4-year-old child had an earache and has been "running a high fever" most of the day. She was seen by the pediatrician yesterday and is taking medication for an infection. The seizure lasted only a few minutes.

    a. What questions should you ask the grandparents regarding the child's medical history?

    _____

    b. What medications should alert you to the likelihood of previous seizures?

    _____

    c. What emergency care is required for this patient?

    _____

40. You are caring for 9-year-old child who lost control of his bicycle while riding down a gravel road. He was thrown over the handlebars and is complaining of severe abdominal pain. He is alert and denies hitting his head or losing responsiveness. Aside from minor scrapes and abrasions, there are no apparent injuries. His mother asks you to immediately transport him to the hospital. You perform initial and focused assessments, immobilize the child on a long backboard with spinal precautions, apply oxygen, and obtain a set of vital signs. His blood pressure is 104/70, pulse rate is 126, and respirations are 22 and shallow.

    a. En route to the hospital, you note that the patient's stomach appears distended. The boy tells you that he feels cold and asks for a blanket. He also says that he is a little sick to his stomach. What do you suspect?

    _____

    b. You repeat his vital signs which are: blood pressure 92/64; pulse rate 130; and respirations 24 and shallow. What does the second set of vital signs suggest to you?

    _____

c. What should you do?

_____

_____

d. The child begins to wretch and vomit. How will you manage his airway?

_____

_____

DIVISION SIX EXAMINATION
INFANTS AND CHILDREN

Directions: Circle the letter of the correct answer.

1. Which age group, developmentally, does not like to be separated from the parents but otherwise tolerates assessment well?
   a. Newborns and infants
   c. Preschool children
   b. Toddlers
   d. School-age children
2. Which age group, developmentally, fears permanent injury, are modest, fears disfigurement, and should be treated as adults?
   a. Toddlers
   c. School-age children
   b. Preschool children
   d. Adolescents
3. Which of the following statements is true?
   a. Infants are obligate nose breathers
   b. A child's tongue is relatively small in comparison with the mouth
   c. Children compensate for respiratory compromise by decreasing their respiratory rate
   d. An infant's airway is less developed and less flexible than an adult's
4. Which of the following statements about oral and nasal airways is true?
   a. The preferred method of inserting an oral airway for a child is by rotating the airway 180° into place
   b. The nasopharyngeal airway is more likely to stimulate vomiting than the oral airway in the child
   c. Nasal airways are useful in children following seizures
   d. The nasal airway only can be inserted into the right nostril
5. Which of the following statements about oxygen delivery for infants and children is true?
   a. Blow-by oxygen means the oxygen is blown directly into the patient's mouth and nose by placing a mask on the patient's face
   b. Parents can be used to assist in delivering oxygen to the patient
   c. Nonrebreather masks should not be used for infants because the oxygen concentration is too high
   d. The flow rate for oxygen delivery via a nonrebreather mask is 4 L/ min in children
6. When ventilating a child patient:
   a. Ventilate the patient until you see a gentle chest rise
   b. The ventilation rate is 30 breaths per minute or one breath every 2 seconds
   c. Use a BVM with a 250 mL bag
   d. Make sure the BVM is equipped with a pop-off valve to reduce gastric distention
7. Which of the following statements about assessing an infant or child is true?
   a. Patients should be considered "V—responsive to voice" in the AVPU categories only if they follow commands
   b. Infants and children generally have mottled skin before they have cyanosis
   c. Capillary refill should take less than 4 seconds if the patient is perfusing adequately
   d. Assess the child patient from the head to trunk, then from toes to trunk
8. Where would you assess the pulse of a responsive 6-month-old patient?
   a. Radial artery
   c. Posterior tibial artery
   b. Carotid artery
   d. Brachial artery

9. EMT–Basics should assess blood pressure for patients older than _____ years of age.
   a. 1   **c.** 3
   b. 2   **d.** 5
10. How should a complete obstruction of the airway be cleared for a responsive 3-year-old child?
    a. Back blows
    b. Abdominal thrusts
    c. Back blows and abdominal thrusts
    d. Back blows and chest thrusts
11. Which of the following is a sign of a complete upper airway obstruction?
    a. The patient is unable to cough
    b. The skin is pink
    c. The patient has expiratory wheezes
    d. The patient has a history of airway disease
12. Which of the following is a sign of early respiratory distress?
    a. Wheezing   **c.** Cyanosis
    b. Limp muscle tone   **d.** Weak or absent distant pulses
13. Which of the following is true:
    a. The patient's response to care provided for a seizure should help the EMT–Basic decide what caused the seizure
    b. Providing good chest compressions is the priority for a near-drowning patient
    c. Altered mental status may be caused by head trauma or infection
    d. Activated charcoal should not be administered to children
14. Which of the following statements is true concerning Sudden Infant Death Syndrome (SIDS)?
    a. SIDS is most common in the third year of life
    b. Do not attempt to resuscitate these patients with basic life-support measures
    c. Question the parents about care and neglect
    d. SIDS deaths do not have an apparent cause or significant history
15. What type of injury is most common in children?
    a. Penetrating trauma   **c.** Burns
    b. Blunt trauma   **d.** Drowning
16. What area of the body is most commonly injured in children?
    a. Head   **c.** Abdomen
    b. Chest   **d.** Extremities
17. What is the most common cause of hypoxia in the unresponsive patient with head injury?
    a. The head injury itself
    b. Failure of EMS personnel to ventilate the patient
    c. The tongue of the patient obstructing the airway
    d. Damage to the trachea
18. Which of the following is true regarding child abuse and neglect?
    a. Neglect is an improper action that injures a child
    b. Physical abuse is more serious than emotional abuse
    c. One sign of abuse are parents who seem inappropriately unconcerned about their child
    d. If abuse is suspected, question the parents at the scene
19. What is the name of the tube placed directly into the stomach for feeding?
    a. Central line   **c.** Gastric tube
    b. Shunt   **d.** Tracheostomy tube

20. Parents are often anxious because:
    a. They do not trust the EMT–Basic caring for their child
    b. They are trying to hide abuse or neglect
    c. They feel helpless
    d. They do not want their child to be treated

DIVISION SEVEN
OPERATIONS

CHAPTER 30
AMBULANCE OPERATIONS

● **CHAPTER OUTLINE**

● MATCHING

Match the terms in Column 1 with the correct definition in Column 2:

Column 1	Column 2
1. _____ Decontamination	a. measures that EMTs take to help prevent the transmission of infection from patients to EMTs, from one patient to another, and from EMTs to patients
2. _____ Disinfectant	b. another emergency vehicle that accompanies the ambulance to the scene or from the scene to the receiving facility
3. _____ Due regard	c. process of killing microorganisms on a surface or item
4. _____ Escort	d. disinfecting process that destroys all microorganisms including bacterial spores
5. _____ Infection control	e. principle that a reasonable and careful person in similar circumstances would act in a way that is safe and considerate for others
6. _____ Sterilization	f. use of physical or chemical means to remove, inactivate, or destroy blood-borne pathogens on a surface or item so that it can no longer transmit infection

● REVIEW QUESTIONS

1. Preparation for the call includes checking availability and readiness of

   _____, _____, and

   _____.

2. Participating in continuing education is also considered part of preparing for a call. **True or false?**

3. List three items of personal protective equipment:

   a. _____

   b. _____

   c. _____

4. Personal protective gear is part of the nonmedical equipment that should be on every ambulance. **True or false?**

5. Dispatch information typically includes the number of patients, their chief complaint, and location. **True or false?**

6. A safe emergency vehicle driver always _____.
   a. Anticipates actions of others
   b. Plans alternative routes for different times of the day
   c. Uses vehicle warning devices wisely
   d. All of the above

7. All drivers respond in a predictable manner when an emergency vehicle approaches. **True or false?**

8. List three factors that contribute to emergency vehicle crashes.

   a. _____

   b. _____

   c. _____

9. En route is also a time to _____.
   a. Discuss the previous call
   b. Get more information from dispatch
   c. Plan for equipment and personal needs
   d. A and B
   e. B and C

10. The first priority in parking at the scene is _____.

11. Arrival at the scene is a good time to _____.
   a. Plan for equipment needs
   b. Reach the patient as soon as possible
   c. Call for additional resources based on scene size-up
   d. Remove all patients immediately to your vehicle

12. Patient transport to a receiving facility is always with lights and siren. **True or false?**

13. The EMT in the patient compartment should use transport time to perform the _____.
   a. Focused history and physical examination
   b. Initial assessment
   c. Detailed and ongoing assessment
   d. Care for life-threatening injuries

14. Patient transfer includes putting the patient in the appropriate room and

    giving _____ report.

15. Documentation can be done after returning to the station. **True or false?**

16. Which type of disinfection is recommended for routine cleaning when no body fluids are present?
   a. High-level disinfection   c. Low-level disinfection
   b. Sterilization   d. Intermediate-level disinfection

17. Which type of disinfection is recommended for equipment that is in contact with areas of the body that are normally sterile?
   a. High-level disinfection   c. Low-level disinfection
   b. Sterilization   d. Intermediate-level disinfection

18. Restocking and rechecking inventory occur during the _____ phase.

19. List three mechanisms of injury that would be possible candidates for air medical transport:

   a. _____

   b. _____

   c. _____

20. Always approach a helicopter from the front, avoiding the pilot's blind areas. **True or false?**

21. You are transporting a cardiac patient to the hospital. His condition stabilized after you applied high-concentration oxygen and assisted him in taking his nitroglycerin. Everything on this call just "seemed to click," and you wish they all could run so smoothly.

a. As part of your preparation for this call, what emergency equipment did you arrange to take to the patient's side while en route to the scene?

_____

_____

_____

b. Your partner carefully drove to the scene with due regard for others. What does due regard require during an emergency response?

_____

_____

_____

c. What are your responsibilities during transfer of this patient at the receiving facility?

_____

_____

_____

CHAPTER 31
GAINING ACCESS

● **CHAPTER OUTLINE**

I. Fundamentals of Extrication

II. Safety and Equipment

A. Personal Safety

B. Patient Safety

C. Other Safety Issues

III. Accessing the Patient

IV. Removing the Patient

163

1. Define the term *extrication*:

_____

2. The role of the incident commander is to _____ efforts of medical and rescue personnel.

3. Extrication requires specialized education and equipment. **True or false?**

4. In all cases of entrapment, _____ _____

   _____ precedes extrication.

5. EMS and rescue personnel should work together to _____.
   a. Remove the patient as quickly as possible
   b. Provide critical interventions
   c. Prepare equipment necessary for immobilization
   d. None of the above

6. Place the following statements about safety during an extrication in order by priority:

   _____ Bystander safety

   _____ Personal safety

   _____ Crew safety

   _____ Patient safety

7. List five pieces of protective gear necessary for extrication:

   a. _____

   b. _____

   c. _____

   d. _____

   e. _____

8. During extrication cover the patient to _____.
   a. Lessen the noise
   b. Protect from debris
   c. Keep the patient from being scared
   d. Keep the patient from being identified

9. Bystanders and onlookers can be helpful during an extrication. **True or false?**

10. List three issues or potential hazards at the scene of an automobile crash:

   a. _____

   b. _____

   c. _____

11. The safety officer is a(n) _____ observer who helps

    identify additional _____ not readily apparent to the EMTs.

12. Define simple and complex access:

    _____

13. List three types of specialized rescue:

    a. _____

    b. _____

    c. _____

14. Which of the following is a reason for extrication prior to spinal immobilization?
    a. The patient has no pain to the neck
    b. The patient cannot be treated in the position he/she is in
    c. The initial assessment revealed no injuries
    d. The patient has no feeling in his/her legs

15. Removing a patient from a vehicle usually requires only two people. **True or false?**

16. You have been dispatched to a helicopter crash. En route you are advised by police on the scene that two victims are trapped in the wreckage. A second ambulance and fire and rescue personnel have also been dispatched.
    a. What is your first priority at this scene?

    _____

    _____

    b. Because you will arrive before fire and rescue personnel, what minimal personal protective equipment should you have available?

    _____

    _____

    c. During scene size-up, you see downed power lines around the wreckage. What should you do?

    _____

    _____

CHAPTER 32

OVERVIEWS: SPECIAL RESPONSE SITUATIONS

● **CHAPTER OUTLINE**

I. Hazardous Materials

    A. Extent of the Problem

    B. Safety Concerns

    C. Approaching the Scene

    D. Information Resources

    E. Procedures

    F. Education for Emergency Medical Services Responders

II. Incident Management Systems

    A. Structure of Responsibilities

    B. Role of the Emergency Medical Technician

III. Multiple Casualty Situations

    A. Triage

    B. Procedures

● MATCHING

Match the terms in Column 1 with the correct definition in Column 2:

Column 1

1. _____ Extrication sector

2. _____ Hazardous material

3. _____ Incident management system

4. _____ Material Safety Data Sheets

5. _____ Placard

6. _____ Staging sector

7. _____ Support or supply sector

8. _____ Transportation sector

9. _____ Treatment sector

10. _____ Triage

11. _____ Triage sector

Column 2

a. information sign with symbols and numbers to assist in identifying the hazardous material or class of material

b. sector in the incident management system responsible for dealing with extrication of patients who are trapped at the scene

c. sector in the incident management system that coordinates with the transportation sector for the movement of vehicles to and from the transportation sector

d. sector of the incident management system that coordinates resources including receiving hospitals, air medical resources, and ambulances

e. system for coordinating procedures to assist in the control, direction, and coordination of emergency response resources

f. sector in the incident management system responsible for obtaining additional resources including disposable supplies, personnel, and equipment for other sectors

g. optional sector in the incident management system that prioritizes patients for treatment and transport

h. any substance or material that can pose an unreasonable risk to health, safety, or property

i. method of categorizing patients into treatment or transport priorities

j. sector in the incident management system that provides care to patients received from the triage and extrication sector

k. information sheets required by the US Department of Labor that list properties and hazards associated with chemicals and compounds to assist in management of incidents involving them

● REVIEW QUESTIONS

1. Hazardous materials scenes only occur at industrial sites. **True or false?**

2. The primary concern at any hazardous material scene is _____.

3. Always approach a hazardous material scene from a(n) _____

   and _____ direction.

4. Container _____ and _____ are helpful in identifying the possible chemical.
   - **a.** Size; color
   - **b.** Shape; texture
   - **c.** Size; shape
   - **d.** Color; texture

5. Always maintain a safe distance and do not enter an unsafe area. **True or false?**

6. Every EMT should be educated to at least the _____ level of hazardous materials knowledge.
   - **a.** First Responder Awareness
   - **b.** First Responder Operations
   - **c.** Hazardous Materials Technicians
   - **d.** Hazardous Materials Specialist

7. List the steps the EMT–Basic should take when approaching a potential hazardous materials scene:

   a. _____

   b. _____

   c. _____

   d. _____

   e. _____

   f. _____

   g. _____

   h. _____

8. List at least three sources of information and assistance with a hazardous material incident.

   a. _____

   b. _____

   c. _____

9. Incident management systems _____. (mark all that apply)
   - **a.** Provide a group leader
   - **b.** Provide an orderly method for communications
   - **c.** Provide unlimited resources
   - **d.** Provide efficient interaction with other agencies
   - **e.** Provide orderly decision making

10. List two situations in which a major incident should be declared:

    a. _____

    b. _____

11. The _____ sector provides care for patients as they are received from triage and extrication.

12. The _____ sector provides resources, supplies, personnel, and equipment.

13. Within each sector there is a _____ _____ that runs the operation of the sector.

14. During a major incident or a mass casualty situation, what should the EMT–Basic who arrives after the incident command system has been established do first?
    a. Report to the triage sector
    b. Begin transporting the most critically ill patients
    c. Begin caring for the most critically injured patients
    d. Report to the staging area for assignment

15. A method of categorizing patient treatment and transport needs is called

    _____.

16. Explain the purpose of triage tags:

    _____

17. Match the patient with the correct priority:
    A = highest; B = second; C = lowest

    _____ Severed artery in leg

    _____ Contusion and laceration to forearm

    _____ Circumferential burn to chest

    _____ Absent pulse and respirations

    _____ Deformity to one wrist with contusions

    _____ Burns to arms, hands, and feet

    _____ Cool, clammy skin, low blood pressure, rapid heart rate

    _____ Pain, swelling, and deformity to thigh

    _____ Severe back and neck pain, motor, sensory functions intact

18. You and your partner have just witnessed a train derailment where multiple patients have been injured. Your department just completed an education program for mass casualty management, and you feel that you are prepared for "the big one." The first step in managing a major incident is to declare that one exists. You advise dispatch and mentally prepare to manage the scene.
    a. Describe situations in which a major incident should be declared.

    _____

    _____

    _____

b. As other emergency services arrive on the scene, you establish EMS sectors. What are seven generally recognized EMS sectors?

_____

_____

_____

c. A person more qualified to manage the incident arrives and assumes command. She assigns you to the triage sector as the triage officer. What are your new responsibilities?

_____

_____

_____

DIVISION SEVEN EXAMINATION
OPERATIONS

Directions: Circle the letter of the correct answer.

1. Which of the following pieces of equipment should be available for EMT–Basics to respond to emergency calls?
   a. Esophageal airways
   c. IV solutions
   b. Splinting supplies
   d. Cardiac medications
2. Which of the following should be routine procedure when en route to the call?
   a. Seatbelts should be secured
   b. Red lights and sirens should be used
   c. Review the specifics of the previous call
   d. All of the above
3. Which of the following is an acceptable method of parking the unit at the scene?
   a. Park downhill from hazards
   c. Park 15 m from any wreckage
   b. Park downwind from hazards
   d. Use emergency lights
4. On arrival at the scene, what should be done?
   a. Notify dispatch of arrival on scene
   b. Size-up scene
   c. Call for additional help if necessary
   d. All the above
5. Which of the following should be performed while en route to the receiving facility?
   a. Begin to care for life-threatening injuries
   b. Ongoing assessment of the patient
   c. Initial assessment of the patient
   d. Ask patient for insurance and billing information
6. When is the verbal patient report given over the radio to the physician or nurse at the receiving facility?
   a. From the scene
   b. While en route to the receiving facility
   c. When arriving at the receiving facility
   d. Report at bedside is sufficient
7. Which of the following pieces of equipment requires high-level disinfection?
   a. Blood pressure cuff
   c. Mask of a bag-valve-mask
   b. Penlights
   d. Dressings
8. Landing zones for EMS helicopters should be _____.
   a. Ideally 30 m by 30 m (100 ft by 100 ft)
   b. Ideally 20 m by 20 m (65 ft by 65 ft)
   c. Minimally 30 m by 30 m (100 ft by 100 ft)
   d. Minimally 12 m by 12 m (40 feet by 40 feet)
9. The EMS helicopter:
   a. Should be approached from the rear (6 o'clock position) for safety
   b. Should be approached from the uphill side for safety
   c. Should be used based on time and injury considerations
   d. Is only used for trauma situations
10. Which of the following is true:
    a. Simple access can still require power tools for patient extrication
    b. Patient safety precedes the safety of crew members once EMT–Basics begin care
    c. Turnout coats and helmets are required for any rescue situation
    d. Patients can be removed from a vehicle crash without spinal precautions if they have no neck or back pain

11. What is the role of the nonrescue EMT–Basic?
   a. Administer care necessary prior to extrication
   b. Work with others who perform rescue
   c. Cooperate with other workers without allowing their activities to interfere with patient care
   d. All the above
12. Chemtrec is:
   a. A manufacturer of chemicals that are not hazardous to people or the environment
   b. A hazardous materials team that responds to major incidents
   c. A reference book listing all chemical placards
   d. A service that provides immediate on-line advice about hazardous materials
13. EMT–Basics should receive education at least to the _____ level for hazardous materials.
   a. First responder operations
   b. First responder awareness
   c. Hazardous materials specialist
   d. Hazardous materials technician
14. Which of the following is true:
   a. Hazardous materials are not found in homes or offices
   b. Park the ambulance upwind from hazardous materials
   c. If no hazardous materials are detected, the scene is safe to enter
   d. Almost every chemical has an odor or color
15. Which of the following sectors of an incident command system is responsible for coordinating available resources of receiving hospitals, air medical services, and ambulances:
   a. Transportation sector
   b. Staging sector
   c. Support sector
   d. Supply sector
16. Triage means:
   a. Sorting patients based on their type of injury or illness (respiratory, cardiac, trauma, etc.)
   b. Categorizing patients based on age
   c. Categorizing patients based on severity of illness or injury
   d. Treating patients based on their injuries
17. During triage, EMT–Basics should:
   a. Splint angulated injuries
   b. Complete an initial assessment and detailed physical examination
   c. Categorize patients based on the type of injury
   d. Correct life-threatening injuries
18. Patients with no pulse or respirations are categorized as:
   a. Highest priority
   b. Intermediate priority
   c. A higher priority than minor burns and cuts
   d. The lowest priority
19. A patient with burns to the face, neck, and throat, with difficulty breathing would be categorized as:
   a. Highest priority
   b. Second priority
   c. The same priority as a patient with major bone injuries
   d. Lowest priority

DIVISION EIGHT
ADVANCED AIRWAY (ELECTIVE)

CHAPTER 33
ADVANCED AIRWAY TECHNIQUES

● **CHAPTER OUTLINE**

I. Sellick Maneuver

   A. Purpose

   B. Anatomic Location

   C. Technique

   D. Special Considerations

II. Advanced Airway Management of Adults

   A. Orotracheal Intubation

      1. Purpose

      2. Indications

      3. Equipment

      4. Techniques of insertion

      5. Complications

   B. Tracheal Suctioning

III. Advanced Airway Management of Children and Infants

   A. Nasogastric Tubes

   B. Orotracheal Intubation

      1. Anatomic and physiological considerations

      2. Indications

      3. Equipment

      4. Techniques of insertion

      5. Complications

● MATCHING

Match the terms in Column 1 with the correct definition in Column 2:

Column 1

1. _____ Apices of the lungs

2. _____ Apneic

3. _____ Bases of the lungs

4. _____ Carina

5. _____ Compliance

6. _____ Direct laryngoscopy

7. _____ Endotracheal tube

8. _____ Epigastrium

9. _____ Extubation

10. _____ Gastric distention

11. _____ Glottic opening

12. _____ Laryngoscope

13. _____ Mainstem bronchi

14. _____ Murphy's eye

15. _____ Nasogastric tube

16. _____ Orotracheal intubation

17. _____ Pulse oximetry

18. _____ Self-extubation

19. _____ Sternal notch

20. _____ Stylet

21. _____ Vallecula

Column 2

a. process of placing an endotracheal tube into the trachea while visualizing the glottic opening with a laryngoscope

b. removal of a tube

c. bendable device placed in the endotracheal tube, giving it rigidity and enabling it to hold a shape

d. term referring to patients who are not breathing

e. process of indirectly measuring the amount of oxygen carried in the blood

f. tube placed into the trachea to increase the delivery of oxygen to the lungs and decrease the possibility of aspiration

g. two branches from the trachea to the lungs

h. anatomic space between the vocal cords, leading to the trachea

i. measure of the elasticity of the lungs

j. tube placed through the nose, down the esophagus, and into the stomach

k. process of inserting an endotracheal tube through the mouth

l. point at which the trachea divides into the two mainstem bronchi

m. bottoms of the lungs, lying approximately at the level of the sixth rib

n. patient's intentional or unintentional removal of a tube

o. tops of the lungs, lying just under the clavicles bilaterally

p. small hole in the side of an endotracheal tube that provides a passage of air if the tip of the tube becomes clogged

q. anatomic location created by the clavicles and the sternum

r. instrument used to visualize the airway during endotracheal intubation

s. anatomic space between the base of the tongue and the epiglottis

t. area over the stomach

u. accumulation of air in the stomach, which places pressure on the diaphragm, making artificial ventilation difficult and increasing the possibility of vomiting

1. What is the purpose of the Sellick maneuver?

_____

_____

2. The proper place to push on the trachea to perform the Sellick maneuver is
   _____.
   a. Adam's apple   c. Thyroid cartilage
   b. Cricoid ring   d. Cricothyroid membrane
3. The Sellick maneuver must be maintained until an endotracheal tube is in position and the position of the tube is confirmed. **True or false?**
4. List four indications for endotracheal intubation:

   a. _____

   b. _____

   c. _____

   d. _____
5. Label the parts of the endotracheal tube on Figure 33-1.

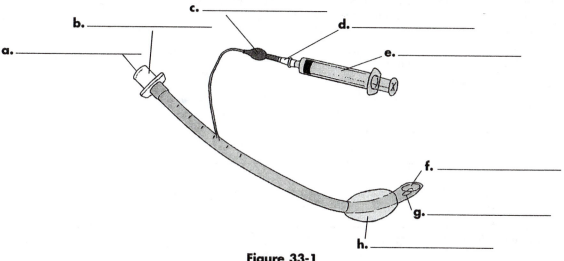

b. _____   **c.** _____   **d.** _____

a. _____   **e.** _____

f. _____

g. _____

h. _____

Figure 33-1

6. Most men require an endotracheal tube between _____, and most women usually require a _____.
   a. 8-9; 6-8   c. 8-10; 6.5-7.5
   b. 8-8.5; 7-8   d. 8.5-9.5; 7.5-8.5
7. List the function of the following:

   Stylet _____

   Pilot balloon _____

   Murphy's eye _____

8. The straight, or _____, blade lifts the epiglottis, whereas the curved or, _____, blade lifts just in front of the epiglottis to help visualize the cords.

9. A commercial device should be used to secure the endotracheal tube in place; tape will not secure the tube adequately. **True or false?**

10. Which of the following is true:
    a. The adult patient's head should be placed in a flexed position when preparing for intubation
    b. The endotracheal tube should be inserted into an adult patient until Murphy's eye just passes the vocal cords
    c. Infants may require a towel to be placed under the upper back to elevate the shoulders
    d. The Sellick maneuver should not be performed on infants prior to intubation

11. Gurgling sounds heard over the epigastrium with ventilation mean the tube is in the _____ and must be removed immediately.
    a. Trachea   c. Esophagus
    b. Right mainstem bronchus   d. Vallecula

12. The absence of breath sounds on the left side of the chest and presence of breath sounds on the right side of the chest after intubation usually means the tube is in the _____.
    a. Stomach   c. Esophagus
    b. Right mainstem bronchus   d. Left mainstem bronchus

13. The maximum amount of time that is allowed for an intubation procedure between ventilations is _____ seconds.
    a. 60   c. 30
    b. 15   d. 45

14. List five complications of intubation:

    a. _____

    b. _____

    c. _____

    d. _____

    e. _____

15. List two indications for tracheal suctioning:

    a. _____

    b. _____

16. A nasogastric tube is indicated for which of the following patients?
    a. A patient with head trauma and without spontaneous respirations
    b. A patient who is apneic with a palpable central pulse
    c. A patient who is alert and responsive with abdominal pain
    d. A patient you are unable to ventilate because of gastric distention

17. Which of the following is true?
    a. The cricoid ring of infants and children become less rigid as they mature
    b. A child's tongue is smaller proportionally than an adult's and takes up less room in the mouth
    c. The cricoid ring is the narrowest portion of the airway in infants and children
    d. The trachea and vocal cords in children are lower and lie more posteriorly than in adults

18. List four indications for endotracheal intubation in an infant or child:

    a. _____

    b. _____

    c. _____

    d. _____

19. The formula used to select an endotracheal tube size for children is:
    a. (16 + age in years) divided by 4
    b. (16 + age in months) divided by 4
    c. (4 + age in years) divided by 16
    d. (4 + age in months) divided by 16

20. What two anatomic structures can be used as alternate methods to determine the size of a child's airway?

    a. _____

    b. _____

21. A slow heart rate in a child is an indication that the patient is receiving adequate amounts of oxygen. **True or false?**

22. Which of the following complications is of greater risk in the infant and child than the adult?
    a. Self-extubation   c. Esophageal intubation
    b. Mainstem intubation   d. The risks are the same

23. Your crew is working a cardiac arrest. The AED has been applied, and three sets of stacked shocks have been delivered. Medical direction advises you to intubate the patient's trachea.
    a. Why is endotracheal intubation indicated and what are the advantages?

    _____

    _____

    b. List the equipment required for intubation.

    _____

    _____

    c. After intubating the patient's trachea, your partner notes diminished lung sounds on the left side. What does this indicate and what should you do to correct it?

    _____

    _____

    _____

Directions: Circle the letter of the correct answer.

1. What is the name of the maneuver performed to prevent passive regurgitation?
   a. Sellick maneuver
   b. Trendelenburg maneuver
   c. Thyroid maneuver
   d. Gastric pressure

2. Which of the following statements best defines the anatomic location of the cricoid ring?
   a. Superior to the cricothyroid membrane
   b. Inferior to the cricothyroid membrane
   c. Superior to the thyroid membrane
   d. Medial to the cricothyroid membrane

3. Which of the following methods would the EMT–Basic use when intubating?
   a. Blind intubation
   b. Retrograde intubation
   c. Digital intubation
   d. Orotracheal intubation

4. Which of the following patients meets the criteria for intubation by an EMT–Basic?
   a. Responsive patient with acute pulmonary edema
   b. Patient who is unresponsive to verbal stimulus but has a gag reflex
   c. An apneic patient who cannot be ventilated with a bag-valve-mask
   d. Responsive patient with difficulty breathing

5. What size endotracheal tube should be used as a rule for emergency intubation of all adult patients?
   a. 7.0 mm i.d.
   b. 7.5 mm i.d.
   c. 8.0 mm i.d.
   d. 8.5 mm i.d.

6. When using the curved blade, what anatomic landmark should be used for its placement?
   a. Vocal cords
   b. Epiglottis
   c. Vallecula
   d. Glottic opening

7. What should be used to lubricate the endotracheal tube?
   a. Water
   b. Vaseline
   c. Water-soluble gel
   d. Tubes should not be lubricated

8. How far into the endotracheal tube should a stylet be inserted?
   a. Approximately 1 inch from the end of the tube
   b. 0.25 inches from the cuff, or proximal end of Murphy's eye
   c. Stylets should not be used for intubation
   d. To the tip of the endotracheal tube

9. Which of the following statements best describes how the blade is inserted into the patient's mouth?
   a. Hold the laryngoscope in your left hand, insert laryngoscope blade into the right corner of the patient's mouth, and lift and sweep the tongue to the left
   b. Hold the laryngoscope in your right hand, insert laryngoscope blade into the left corner of the patient's mouth, and lift and sweep the tongue to the right
   c. Hold the laryngoscope in your left hand, insert laryngoscope blade into the left corner of the patient's mouth, and lift and sweep the tongue to the left
   d. Hold the laryngoscope in your left hand, insert laryngoscope blade into the middle of the patient's mouth, and lift and sweep the tongue to the left or right

10. How much air should be inserted in the cuff of the endotracheal tube in the adult patient?
    a. 3-5 cc c. 10-20 cc
    b. 5-10 cc d. 30 cc
11. What location should be auscultated first following insertion of the endotracheal tube?
    a. Left base c. Sternal notch
    b. Right base d. Epigastrium
12. If no sounds are heard over the lung fields and gurgling is heard over the stomach, the EMT–Basic should:
    a. Ventilate the patient 12 times per minute
    b. Put more air in the cuff of the endotracheal tube and listen again
    c. Deflate the cuff and remove the tube
    d. Pull back on the endotracheal tube until breath sounds are heard
13. If the tube is placed in the right main stem bronchus, what action should the EMT–Basic take?
    a. Deflate the cuff and slowly pull the tube back until breath sounds are heard in all lung fields
    b. Put more air in the cuff of the endotracheal tube and listen again
    c. Deflate the cuff, remove the tube, hyperventilate the patient for 2 to 3 minutes, and attempt to intubate again
    d. Remove the tube, ventilate the patient, and do not attempt to reintubate the patient
14. Where should the cuff of a properly placed endotracheal tube lie?
    a. At the carina c. Just past the vocal cords
    b. Superior to the epiglottis d. At the sternal notch
15. Which of the following is NOT a complication of intubation?
    a. Esophageal intubation c. Soft-tissue damage
    b. Bradycardia d. Damage to the alveoli
16. Which catheter should be used to suction the nasopharynx or inside the endotracheal tube?
    a. Rigid catheter c. Just the suction tube with no catheter
    b. Tonsil tip catheter d. Soft catheter
17. Which of the following devices is used to decompress the stomach?
    a. Endotracheal tube c. Nasogastric tube
    b. Foley tube d. Nasopharyngeal tube
18. Which laryngoscope blade is preferred when intubating an infant?
    a. A curved blade c. A straight blade
    b. A MacIntosh blade d. No particular blade is preferred
19. What is the formula used to determine the tube size for an infant or child patient?
    a. (16 + age in years) divided by 4
    b. (18 + age in years) divided by 4
    c. (16 + age in months) divided by 6
    d. (4 + age in years) divided by 4
20. Which of the following is a unique feature of pediatric endotracheal tubes?
    a. The size is not indicated
    b. There are one or more black rings on the distal end
    c. Infant tubes take more air in the cuff
    d. Murphy's hole is in the other side of the tube

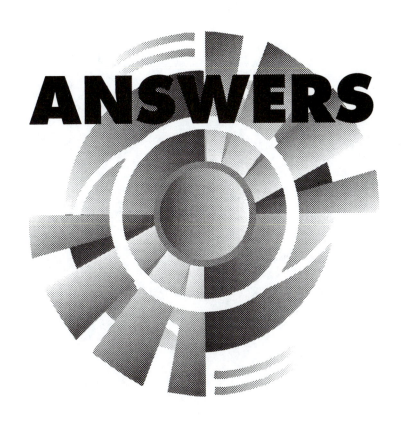

ANSWERS

CHAPTER 1
INTRODUCTION TO EMERGENCY MEDICAL CARE

MATCHING

1. F
2. G
3. A
4. E
5. L
6. K
7. H
8. J
9. D
10. B
11. I
12. C

Definitions to key terms can be found on page 3 of the student textbook. Key terms cover Objectives 1, 2, and 6.

REVIEW QUESTIONS

1. False. Universal access is not one of NHTSA's 10 standards for EMS. The 10 standards include: Regulation and policy; Resource management; Human resources and education; Transportation; Facilities; Communications; Public information and education; Medical direction; Trauma systems; and Evaluation. p. 5, Objective 1

2. True. The facilities standard helps EMS systems make decisions about what is the closest appropriate facility for any particular patient, such as a Children's hospital for a pediatric patient. p. 6, Objective 1

3. D. First responders should provide initial stabilization until additional EMS resources arrive. The first responder course is designed for persons who are likely to encounter an ill or injured patient in their job but who are not educated for ambulance service. First responders generally stabilize the patient until more help arrives. EMT–Intermediates and –Paramedics are often taught advanced care for trauma patients and to start IVs and administer medications. p. 7, Objective 2

4. C. The EMT–Basic course prepares people to manage life-threatening injuries and illnesses. p. 7, Objective 2

5. There are many ways to help ensure personal safety, including: maintaining a healthy body; remaining physically fit; using body substance isolation precautions; and sizing-up the scene for potential hazards. p. 9, Objective 3

6. False. EMT–Basics are responsible for their own personal safety, the safety of their crew members, the patient, and bystanders. EMT–Basics may work with other EMS personnel to ensure the safety of the scene and everyone involved. p. 10, Objective 4

7. Roles and responsibilities of the EMT–Basic include: Personal safety; Safety of the crew, patient, and bystanders; Patient assessment and care; Lifting and moving patients; Transport and transfer of care; and Patient advocacy. p. 10, Objective 2

8. D. Professional appearance and manner will help reduce the anxiety of the patient and the family. A clean uniform, neat appearance, and confident manner are all a part of being professional. p. 11

9. C. A medical director is a physician who monitors the care given to patients by EMT–Basics. Medical directors function on- and off-line. p. 12, Objective 6

10. True. Direct, or on-line, medical direction refers to physicians talking with EMT–Basics in the field, face-to-face, or over the radio or telephone. p. 12, Objective 6

11. Quality improvement is a system of internal/ external reviews and audits of all aspects of an EMS system to identify those aspects needing improvement. p. 12, Objective 5

12. D. All of the definitions listed describe medical direction. p. 12, Objective 6

13. **a.** Roles and responsibilities of the EMT–Basic include: personal safety; safety of the crew, patient, and bystanders; patient assessment; patient care based on assessment findings; lifting and moving patients safely; transport and transfer of care; record keeping and data collection; and patient advocacy (patient rights). p. 9. **b.** An EMS response includes: emergency recognition; system access; EMS personnel dispatch and response; care provided to the patient at the scene; medical direction when necessary; patient stabilization, transportation, and delivery to the hospital. p. 5. **c.** By dialing 9-1-1 or a 7-digit phone number (in areas that do not have 9-1-1 access). p. 7

CHAPTER 2
THE WELL-BEING OF THE EMT–BASIC

MATCHING

1. D
2. B
3. C
4. E
5. A

Definitions to key terms can be found on page 17 of the student textbook. Key terms cover Objectives 5, 6, and 8.

6. 2—anger; 3—bargaining; 1—denial; 5—acceptance; 4—depression. p. 18, Objective 2

7. 3—the patient; 1—personal safety; 4—bystander safety; 2—other crew members; p. 23, Objective 7

● REVIEW QUESTIONS

1. False. People move through the stages of death and dying at their own rate. Some people skip stages, and some people never work through all of the stages. p. 18, Objective 2

2. EMT–Basics can help the family members of a dying patient by listening to their concerns without falsely reassuring them that the patient will get better. Tell the family members that everything possible is being done for the patient. Allow family members to stay with the patient if possible, and allow them to express their emotions. p. 19, Objective 3

3. A. To reduce stress: change your diet; stop smoking; get regular exercise; learn to relax; balance work; enjoy recreation and family; change work schedule; and seek professional help. p. 20, Objective 3

4. True. EMT–Basics may have emotional reactions such as irritability, anxiety, indecisiveness, guilt, or depression as a reaction to stress. Feelings such as guilt may occur even when the EMT–Basic cares for the patient to the best of his/her ability. p. 20, Objective 6

5. Any situation can cause stress for an EMT–Basic. Situations that are likely to cause stress include: mass casualty incidents; infant and child trauma; traumatic amputation; infant or child, spouse, or elder abuse; death or injury of a co-worker or other public safety personnel; and emergency response to the illness or injury of a friend or family member. p. 20, Objective 5

6. Stress can be caused by: *physical, chemical,* or *emotional* factors. p. 20, Objective 5

7. Warning signs of stress include: irritability with co-workers, family, friends, and patients; inability to concentrate; physical exhaustion; difficulty sleeping or nightmares; anxiety; indecisiveness; guilt; loss of appetite; loss of interest in sexual activities; isolation; loss of interest in work; increased substance use or abuse; and depression. p. 20, Objective 5

8. True. Stress can build up over time or occur as a result of a single critical incident. p. 22, Objective 5

9. True. CISD allows people to talk over their fears and feelings, helping to speed up the recovery process. p. 22, Objective 5

10. False. Family members of EMT–Basics often face stress related to the EMS profession. Stress is caused by not understanding the profession; by the inability to plan family events because of on-call shifts, rotating shifts, and late ambulance calls; and by the fear of injury on the job. p. 22, Objective 4

11. A. Critical incident stress occurs when the EMT–Basic is unable to function in the job due to unusually strong emotional reactions. The other three signs listed are associated with stress, but the EMT–Basic is not necessarily unable to function in the job because of them. p. 22, Objective 5

12. False. Scene safety is the highest priority for an EMT–Basic in every situation and should be assessed before entering the scene or beginning any patient care. p. 23, Objective 7

13. A. Gloves are the only BSI precaution needed when there is minimal bleeding. A mask, protective eyewear, and gown may be necessary anytime the bleeding becomes more severe. Many EMS professionals make a habit of always taking BSI precautions, including wearing protective eyewear. p. 26, Objectives 8, 9

14. True. Anytime there is a chance of splashing fluids, the eyes, nose, and mouth should be covered. p. 26, Objectives 8, 9

15. C. EMT–Basics should not enter hazardous materials scenes or treat contaminated patients unless they have undergone specialized hazardous materials education or a specialized hazardous materials crew has made the scene safe. p. 27, Objective 10

16. B. Rescue situations require EMT–Basics to wear protective clothing to prevent injury from sharp metal, glass, etc. Hazardous materials require varying levels of protective clothing. This type of protective clothing is not required for routine emergency calls. p. 28, Objective 10

17. a. The stages of death and dying are: denial; anger; bargaining; depression; and acceptance. Not all people will go through all the stages or go through them in order. p. 18. b. The wife is in the bargaining stage. p. 18. c. Listen to their concerns but do not falsely reassure them. Let them know that everything possible is being done to help. Allow the family members to remain with the patient and to express their feelings and provide comfort measure. p. 19

18. a. Warning signs of stress include: irritability with coworkers, family, friends, or patients; inability to concentrate; physical exhaustion; difficulty sleeping or having nightmares; anxiety; indecisiveness; guilt; loss of appetite; loss of interest in sexual activities; isolation; loss of interest in work; increased substance use or abuse; and depression. p. 20. b. Stress reduction techniques include: changing your diet; quitting smoking; getting regular exercise; learning to relax; balancing work, recreation, and family; changing your work schedule; and seeking professional help. p. 20. c. Any situation can cause stress. The following is a list of situations that commonly cause stress: mass casualty incidents; infant and child trauma; traumatic amputation; infant, child, or elder abuse; death or

injury of a co-worker or other public safety personnel; and an emergency response to the Illness or injury of a friend or family member. p. 20

● CHAPTER 3
MEDICAL/LEGAL AND ETHICAL ISSUES

● MATCHING

1. G
2. I
3. H
4. J
5. E
6. F
7. D
8. C
9. B
10. A

Definitions to key terms can be found on page 33 of the student textbook. Key terms cover Objectives 1, 2, 3, 4, and 7.

● REVIEW QUESTIONS

1. A. In most states, the Department of Transportation National Highway Traffic Safety Administration's National Standard Curriculum is the basis for the scope of practice for EMT–Basics. Medical directors and state legislation may have the ability to limit or expand the scope of practice but generally do not create the basis for the scope of practice. p. 35, Objective 1

2. False. Protocols and standing orders are used to expand the EMT–Basic's scope of practice and allow for greater flexibility in the treatment of patients. p. 35, Objective 1

3. Duty to act means that an EMT–Basic has a legal responsibility to provide emergency medical care when called on or presented with an opportunity to do so. Duty to act can involve a legal consideration (either formal or implied) or an informal obligation. In some states, being licensed or certified means that you have been educated to assist in an emergency and will do so when necessary. p. 36, Objective 8

4. There are four criteria that must be met for negligence to be proven. The EMT–Basic must have a duty to act; there must be a breach of that duty to act; damage must occurr to the patient; and the damage that occurs must be due to the EMT–Basic's actions or inactions, known as proximate cause. p. 37, Objective 7

5. B. EMT–Basics must ensure that the patient's care is continued at the same level or at a higher level to avoid abandonment. An EMT–Basic releasing a patient to hospital staff is the only example listed

of care being transferred to a higher level. p. 37, Objective 7

6. The term that describes permission to be treated is called *consent*. Consent must be given by all competent patients before an EMT–Basic can begin treatment. p. 38, Objective 3

7. False. Parents, as their children's legal guardians, have the right to accept or refuse care on behalf of the child, regardless of the child's wishes. p. 39, Objective 5

8. EMT–Basics should try to persuade a patient who is refusing care to accept treatment, or at least transport for evaluation at the receiving facility. EMT–Basics must inform the patient of the risks associated with refusing treatent and transport. After ensuring the patient is competent to refuse, contact medical direction and then properly document the patient's refusal. Be sure to inform the patient that you will be willing to return if the patient changes his/her mind, and document this also. p. 40, Objective 6

9. C. Assault occurs when someone is threatened with offensive physical contact. Battery occurs when someone is actually touched without consent. Assault and battery are often used interchangeably, but they do have separate definitions. Negligence occurs when an EMT–Basic fails to act as a reasonable, prudent EMT–Basic would under similar circumstances. p. 41, Objective 7

10. True. Advance directives allow a patient's wishes to be known concerning medical treatment in specific situations if the patient is unable to speak for him/herself. p. 42, Objective 2

11. Patient confidentiality is an important concept for EMT–Basics to understand and comply with to protect a patient's right to privacy. EMT–Basics can release confidential information when giving a report to other healthcare workers who will be taking care of the patient, when there is a reportable situation (such as suspected child abuse or gunshot wounds), for third-party payment for service, and when subpoenaed for information by a court of law. p. 44, Objective 9

12. C. Motor vehicle crashes do not routinely require special reports. Neglect, rape, gunshot wounds, stab wounds, animal bites, and certain communicable diseases routinely require reporting. p. 45, Objective 12

13. False. Patients must sign a legal document stating that they wish to donate their organs on dying. EMT–Basics will treat organ donor patients with the same life-saving measures as any other patient. p. 45, Objective 10

14. False. Although EMT–Basics should disturb as little as possible at the crime scene, it may be impossible to treat the patient properly without disturbing the scene. The EMT–Basic should provide all

treatments necessary and note any movement of evidence. p. 46, Objective 11

15. **a.** The standard of care is the minimum acceptable level of care normally provided in the area. p. 35. **b.** Negligence occurs when a patient suffers damage or injury because an EMT fails to perform to the accepted standard of care. p. 37. **c.** For negligence to be proven, four criteria must be met: there was a duty to act; there was a breach of duty; damage occurred; and there was proximate cause. p. 37

16. **a.** Because the patient is unresponsive and unable to give expressed consent, permission to treat would be implied in the scenario. p. 39. **b.** Implied consent assumes that all unresponsive patients suffering from an immediately life-threatening or disabling injury or illness would want to receive treatment and would provide expressed consent if they could. p. 39. **c.** Expressed consent means the patient directly agrees to accept your treatment and gives permission to proceed with care. The patient must be of legal age and able to make a rational decision and must understand the procedure and any associated risks. p. 38

17. **a.** A living will is a type of advance directive that describes the kind of life-saving treatment that a patient wants (or does not want) if the patient becomes unable to request or refuse that treatment. p. 42. **b.** Durable Power of Attorney is a written document identifying a guardian to make medical decisions for the patient when the patient can no longer make these decisions. p. 42. **c.** You should continue with life-support measures, ask the son to produce the written documents, and consult with medical direction. The documents should bear the patient's and witnesses' signatures and should be notarized. p. 43

● CHAPTER 4
THE HUMAN BODY

● MATCHING
1. H
2. N
3. C
4. M
5. A
6. F
7. G
8. B
9. T
10. I
11. U
12. V
13. L
14. R
15. P
16. K
17. D
18. S
19. Q
20. W
21. O
22. J
23. E

Definitions to key terms can be found on page 51 of the student textbook. Key terms cover Objectives 1 and 2.

24. **a.** Lateral; **b.** Posterior; **c.** Midaxillary line; **d.** Superior; **e.** Anterior; **f.** Inferior; **g.** Medial; **h.** Midline. p. 54, Objective 1

25. **a.** Vertebral column; **b.** Ribs; **c.** Radius; **d.** Skull; **e.** Mandible; **f.** Clavicle; **g.** Sternum; **h.** Humerus; **i.** Pelvis; **j.** Femur; **k.** Patella; **l.** Tibia. p. 64, Objective 2

● REVIEW QUESTIONS

1. A. The midaxillary line runs through the armpits and ankles, dividing the body into front and back halves, or anterior and posterior planes. p. 53, Objective 1

2. D. The oropharynx is directly behind the mouth. The nasopharynx is directly behind the nose. The epiglottis is a leaflike flap that prevents food from entering the trachea. The larynx is just below the epiglottis, at the opening of the trachea. p. 53, Objective 2

3. A. The trachea is also known as the windpipe. p. 53, Objective 2

4. C. The diaphragm and the intercostal muscles are used during normal breathing. The diaphragm flattens and lowers when the muscle fibers contract, causing air to be pulled into the lungs. Intercostal muscles contract, causing the ribs to move upward and outward. p. 57, Objective 2

5. B. When the muscle fibers in the diaphragm contract, the dome of the diaphragm flattens and lowers, drawing air into the lungs. p. 57, Objective 2

6. B. The heart consists of four chambers—two atria and two ventricles. p. 60, Objective 2

7. B. Oxygen-poor blood enters the right atrium and is pumped into the right ventricle. The blood is then pumped to the lungs, where it is oxygenated. Blood returns from the lungs into the left atrium, to the left ventricle and then is pumped to the body. p. 60, Objective 2

8. D. Arteries carry blood away from the heart, and veins return blood to the heart. The aorta is an example of an artery. Venules are tiny veins, and capillaries are the smallest blood vessels in the body. p. 61, Objective 2

9. B. The average adult man has 5 to 6 L of blood in his body. p. 61, Objective 2

10. A. The first number recorded in the blood pressure is the systolic pressure, which is the pressure in the arteries when the heart contracts. The second number is the diastolic pressure, which is the pressure in the arteries when the heart is at rest. p. 62, Objective 2

11. Smooth muscle is located in (b) the stomach and intestines. Skeletal muscle (c) attaches to the bone. Cardiac muscle is located in (a) the heart. p. 68, Objective 2

12. A. The central nervous system consists of the brain and spinal cord. The peripheral nervous system consists of the sensory and motor nerves. p. 69, Objective 2

13. True. The peripheral nerves carry sensory and motor information between the spinal column and the other parts of the body, relaying information from the environment to the brain and commands from the brain to the body. p. 69, Objective 2

14. True. Signals are sent to the motor nerves from the brain to the body. The motor nerves cause the skeletal muscles to react and are responsible for the movement of the body. p. 69, Objective 2

15. A. The skin has three layers: the epidermis is the outermost layer; the dermis is the deeper layer containing the sweat glands, hair follicles, blood vessels and nerve endings; and the subcutaneous layer is the deepest layer which stores fat and serves as insulation for the body. p. 70, Objective 2

16. The digestive system breaks down food so that it can be absorbed into the blood and delivered to the cells as nutrients, vitamins, and minerals. p. 70, Objective 2

17. Chemicals released from glands within the body are called *hormones*. Hormones are chemicals released into the blood stream that regulate many of the body's activities. p. 72, Objective 2

18. a. The trachea splits into two main-stem bronchi. The bronchi subdivide into smaller and smaller air passages until they end at the alveoli. p. 56. b. The process of ventilation uses two main sets of muscles: the diaphragm and intercostal muscles, which increase the size of the thoracic cavity, pulling air into the lungs. Exhalation begins with relaxation of these muscles, which decreases the size of the thoracic cavity, forcing air out through the nose and mouth. p. 57. c. As oxygen-rich air enters the alveoli, blood with low levels of oxygen and high levels of carbon dioxide is flowing through the capillaries surrounding the alveoli. Gases move from areas of greater concentration to areas of lesser concentration, and therefore oxygen enters the blood and carbon dioxide is removed. p. 58

19. a. Blood pressure is the measurement of the pressure exerted against the walls of the arteries. It is measured in millimeters of mercury (mm Hg). p. 62. b. The top number is known as the systolic reading, which is the measurement of the pressure pushing against the arterial walls when the heart contracts. The bottom number is the diastolic reading, which is the measurement of the pressure against the arterial walls when the heart relaxes. p. 62. c. You should advise the woman that blood pressure readings can be affected by age and various individual factors. You also should tell her that the measurement of 184/96 is considered higher than average but may be normal for her. She should make an appointment with her private physician to have her blood pressure evaluated more thoroughly. p. 62

20. a. What are skeletal muscles? p. 67. b. What is the peripheral nervous system? p. 69. c. What is the dermis? p. 70

● CHAPTER 5
BASELINE VITAL SIGNS
AND SAMPLE HISTORY

● MATCHING
1. G
2. B
3. C
4. R
5. I
6. S
7. Q
8. A
9. N
10. P
11. E
12. O
13. F
14. H
15. L
16. K
17. J
18. M
19. D

Definitions to key terms can be found on page 77 of the student textbook. Key terms cover Objectives 1, 4, 20, 21, and 24.

● REVIEW QUESTIONS

1. When assessing breathing, assess the rate and *quality* of the patient's respirations. Rate, how often the patient breathes, is expressed in breaths per minute. Quality is measured by assessing depth, use of accessory muscles, and any noises from the airway. p. 79, Objective 3

2. D. The average respiratory rate for an adult is 12 to 20 per minute, for children 15 to 30 per minute, and for infants 25 to 50 per minute. p. 79, Objective 3

3. The respiratory rate is determined by counting the number of breaths in 30 seconds and multiplying by two. If the breathing is irregular, you may need to assess for a full minute. p. 79, Objective 2

4. False. The noise made by the tongue partially blocking the airway is called *snoring*. Crowing is a long, high-pitched sound when breathing in. Both cases indicate a respiratory problem. p. 80, Objective 4

5. False. Pulses can be felt in the arteries when the heart contracts, but not in the veins. Assess pulses in areas when the arteries pass over a bone and close to the skin. p. 80, Objective 5

6. When assessing the pulse, note the *rate* and *quality*. The rate is determined by counting the beats in 30 seconds and multiplying by two. Assessing quality includes determining the regularity and strength of the beats. p. 82, Objectives 5, 6

7. A. The average resting pulse rate for an adult should be 60 to 80. This number is only an average, and rates outside of the average may be normal for a patient. p. 81, Objective 6

8. A regular pulse means that the length of time between each beat is constant. An irregular pulse means there is not a constant time between beats. A weak pulse means that the heart is not pumping effectively or there is low blood volume. p. 81, Objective 7

9. C. When assessing the skin, assess the color, temperature, and condition of the skin. Capillary refill may be assessed in infants and children. p. 82, Objective 8

10. When assessing skin color in the nail beds, oral mucosa, or conjunctiva, the normal skin color is pink, and abnormal skin colors include *flushed* or red, *cyanotic* or blue-gray, *jaundiced* or yellow, and pale. p. 82, Objectives 8, 9, 10

11. To identify skin temperature, the skin of the *trunk* is more reliable than the skin of the extremities. The extremities will become cool faster than the rest of the body and may not be an accurate assessment. p. 82, Objectives 8, 11

12. Abnormal skin temperatures include hot (which may be due to fever or exposure to heat), cool (which may be due to poor perfusion or exposure to cold), and cold (when the patient is exposed to extreme cold). p. 82, Objectives 8, 12

13. B. The normal skin condition is dry. Abnormal skin conditions include moist, wet, and extremely dry. Cool and moist skin is called *clammy skin*. p. 82, Objectives 8, 13

14. B. Capillary refill in infants and children should take less than 2 seconds. A longer time may indicate poor perfusion. p. 83, Objective 8, 14

15. *Dilated* pupils are big, and *constricted* pupils are small. p. 83, Objectives 16, 17

16. Equal and reactive to light means that both pupils constrict when a light is shined into them and that they constrict and dilate equally in relationship to one another. p. 83, Objectives 16, 18

17. C. When pupils react normally to light, they should constrict equally. p. 83, Objectives 16, 18

18. If the light in a room is too bright, the pupils may not react when a light is shined into them. In this case, cover the eyes from light and then expose them to light again to measure the reaction. p. 83, Objective 15

19. True. Blood pressure is a measure of the force exerted against the walls of the arteries, both when the heart is contracting (systolic pressure) and at rest (diastolic pressure). p. 85, Objective 20

20. Blood pressure can be measured by listening using a stethoscope, called *auscultation*, or by feeling for the return of a pulse, called *palpation*. p. 85, Objectives 22, 19

21. D. Stable patients should be assessed every 15 minutes, and unstable patients should be assessed every 5 minutes. Be sure to record this information and include the information in the report to the receiving facility. p. 85, Objectives 22, 19

22. True. SAMPLE stands for Signs/Symptoms, Allergies, Medications, Past pertinent history, Last oral intake, and Events leading to the illness or injury. p. 86, Objective 23

23. False. When assessing a patient's SAMPLE, assess only the patient's pertinent past medical history. p. 86, Objective 23

24. False. A medical identification tag may alert you to information regarding the patient's history, medications, or allergies that would cause you to care for the patient differently. When patients are unable to give you information about themselves, always look for medical identification tags. p. 86, Objective 26

25. It is important to accurately record the vital signs and patient history because trends in the patient's condition may be noted by comparing sets of vital signs. The patient's condition may cause medical direction to direct you to change your care. The history and vital signs also will be valuable information for the personnel at the receiving facility when they begin to decide how they will treat the patient. p. 87, Objective 25

26. **a.** 30-40/min. p. 79. **b.** 80-120 beats/min. p. 79. **c.** 94/54. p. 79

27. **a.** Evaluate the rate and quality of the patient's respirations. p. 79. **b.** Intercostal muscles, neck muscles, chest muscles, abdominal muscles, and upper and lower back muscles are often used as accessory muscles. p. 80. **c.** Wheezing is a high-pitched whistling sound that is usually caused by constriction of smaller airways. p. 80

● CHAPTER 6
LIFTING AND MOVING PATIENTS

● MATCHING

1. D
2. A
3. C
4. F
5. B
6. E

Definitions to key terms can be found on page 91 of the student textbook. Key terms cover Objectives 1 and 10.

● REVIEW QUESTIONS

1. False. It is important to know both your and your partner's lifting capabilities. Call for additional help when necessary. p. 92, Objective 2

2. To lift safely, keep your back straight and use your legs, not your back to lift the patient. Keep the weight close to your body. Call for additional help if necessary. Do not twist your torso when lifting, and keep your feet shoulder width apart. p. 92, Objectives 2, 3

3. False. When possible, roll rather than carry a patient. There are times, however, when carrying the patient is preferable, such as when the terrain is uneven. p. 93, Objective 4

4. False. One-handed carrying techniques allow more rescuers to carry the weight and allow for better balance of the weight. p. 95, Objective 5

5. When it is necessary to carry a patient down stairs, use the stair chair whenever possible. The stair chair is more maneuverable and was designed to carry patients down stairs. The stair chair cannot be used if the patient is unresponsive or has a suspected spinal injury. p. 95, Objective 6

6. B. When possible, do not reach far in front of you or reach for long periods of time. When reaching, keep your back in a locked position, avoid leaning back over your hips, and avoid twisting your back. p. 95, Objective 7

7. When performing a log roll, keep your back straight while leaning over the patient, lean from the hips, and use your shoulder muscles to help with the roll. p. 97, Objective 8

8. A. When possible, push the weight rather than pull. Pushing causes less strain on your body than pulling. p. 95, Objective 9

9. Although there is no time to immobilize the patient when an emergency move is required, the *spine* can be protected by pulling against the long axis of the body. p. 96, Objective 10

10. B. Emergency moves are used when there is a danger to the patient or the rescue crew. p. 96, Objectives 10, 11

11. True. Although the patient should be moved rapidly during an urgent move, take time to protect the spine if there is suspected injury. p. 98, Objective 10

12. The long backboard is used to (b) immobilize the entire patient. The scoop stretcher is used to (a) lift from a supine position to the stretcher. The stair chair is used to (c) move patients through narrow halls or down stairs. The basket stretcher is used as a (e) rescue device. The short backboard is used for (d) immobilization during extrication. p. 103, Objectives 10,12

13. A. A pregnant patient should be rolled onto her left side to prevent the fetus from compressing the vena cava. p. 105, Objective 10

14. False. Any patient with a suspected spinal injury should be fully immobilized on a long backboard. p. 105, Objective 10

15. C. A patient with signs and symptoms of shock should be transported in the shock position, on his/her back with the legs elevated 8 to 12 inches. p. 105, Objective 10

16. A. All patients (except those who are unresponsive or have suspected spinal injuries) should be transported in the position of comfort. p. 105, Objective 10

17. **a.** A stair chair is the best method to use when you must carry a responsive patient down steep stairs. p. 95. **b.** A stair chair should not be used for any patient with a possible spinal injury or who is unresponsive. p. 95. **c.** A patient with a possible spinal injury should be transported down stairs immobilized on a long spine board. p. 95

18. **a.** After ensuring scene safety, you should provide manual stabilization of the cervical spine; open the airway by the jaw-thrust maneuver; clear the airway with suction as needed, and seal the open chest wound. p. 98. **b.** Yes. He is unresponive, has inadequate breathing, and needs life-saving care. p. 98. **c.** One EMT maintains spinal stabilization, while another EMT applies the cervical spine immobilization device and short backboard (wooden or vest type) and supports the torso. A long backboard is placed near the door. The patient is rotated in several short, coordinated moves and lowered onto the backboard. The patient's neck and back are moved as one unit. p. 98

● DIVISION ONE EXAMINATION

1. D. EMT–Basics provide primary care for life-threatening illnesses and injuries before the patient reaches the hospital. First responders stabilize the patient until the ambulance arrives. EMT–Paramedics are advanced-level prehospital

care providers. Definitive care for trauma patients cannot be provided in the prehospital setting. p. 7, Objective 2

2. B. One role of the EMT–Basic is to be an advocate for the patient's rights. EMT–Basics often work with other public safety personnel, including firefighters and police officers. EMT–Basics should be concerned with their personal safety, then the safety of their crew members, followed by the safety of the patient, and then that of the bystanders. All healthcare providers require continuing education to keep their skills current and stay informed about the latest changes in healthcare. p. 8, Objectives 1, 2

3. D. EMT–Basics provide care based on assessment findings, not on a diagnosis. Roles and responsibilities include personal safety; safety of the crew, patient, and bystanders; patient assessment and care; lifting and moving patients; transport and transfer of care; and patient advocacy. p. 10, Objectives 2, 3, 4

4. A. Scene and personal safety must be the first priority during any emergency call. None of the other aspects of patient care can occur if the EMT–Basic is injured. p. 9, Objective 3

5. C. Physician medical directors should be involved in all aspects of emergency medicine, including education, quality improvement, development of protocols and standing orders, and patient treatment decisions. p. 12, Objective 6

6. D. Dying patients or their families may experience Denial, Anger, Bargaining, Depression, and Acceptance. Not all patients and their families go through all of the stages, or they may not go through them in order. Sympathy is not a stage of death and dying. p. 18, Objective 2

7. A. Respect the patient's needs for dignity, sharing, communications, privacy and control. Do not lie or falsely reassure the patient or the family for any reason. Be honest and direct when answering their questions. When appropriate, a reassuring touch can console and comfort the patient and the family members. Allow the patient to remain near family members when possible. p. 19, Objectives 2, 3

8. D. CISD is an acronym for Critical Incident Stress Debriefing, which is a process to help emergency workers deal with emotions and stresses caused by on-the-job responsibilities. p. 22, Objective 6

9. D. Critical incident stress debriefing includes preincident stress education, on-scene peer support, support for families of emergency workers, and follow up-care for emergency workers. p. 22, Objective 6

10. C. Surgical masks (worn by the patient of the EMT–Basic) or HEPA respirators (worn by the EMT–Basic) can be used by EMT–Basics when necessary as part of their body substance isolation precautions. Some masks have eye protection shields attached. Self-contained breathing apparatus may be used in some situations but are not routinely included in body substance isolation precautions from blood and other body fluids. Industrial grade goggles and helmets with chin straps are used for rescue operations. p. 24, Objective 10

11. B. Negligence occurs when a patient suffers damages or injury because of the EMT–Basics actions or inactions. Abandonment occurs when care is not continued at the same or higher level. Assault and/or battery occurs when a patient is treated without his/her consent or after refusing treatment. p. 37, Objective 7

12. B. Patients who are unresponsive can be treated under the terms of implied consent. A patient must be responsive to give expressed consent. Parents have the right to refuse care for their children, and EMT–Basics must honor this refusal. Patients have the right to change their mind and refuse care even after initially giving consent. p. 38, Objectives 3, 4, 5

13. D. When you are not sure if a patient should be treated or not, err on the side of treatment. When a patient refuses care, the EMT–Basic must explain why care is needed and explain the potential risks involved with refusing treatment. Contact medical direction and have the patient and a witness sign a refusal form. Patients have the right to refuse or withdraw from treatment any time. Parents can make decisions regarding the care of their child, even if the child refuses. p. 40, Objectives 3, 4, 5

14. A. Patients have the right to decide, along with their physicians, what treatment plan is best for them in the event that they cannot speak for themselves. Some states do not recognize the DNR as being within the scope of practice for prehospital care providers. The DNR order must be signed by the physician and the patient and must be seen by the EMT–Basic at the scene. p. 42, Objective 2

15. C. Confidential information can be released when the patient is involved in a reportable situation, such as child abuse. EMT–Basics should take care not to divulge confidential information when using a case for continuing education. EMT–Basics can give confidential information to law enforcement personnel when subpoenaed. p. 44, Objective 9

16. A. The pharynx is another word for the throat. The olecranon process is part of the upper extremity. The mitral valve is in the heart to prevent the backflow of blood from the left ventricle to the left atrium. Adrenalin is a hormone that helps prepare the body for emergencies. p. 67, Objective 2

17. C. The trachea of an infant or child is more easily obstructed by swelling or foreign objects due to the smaller size. In general, all of the structures of

the respiratory system in children are smaller and more easily obstructed. The tongue is large and often causes obstruction. The trachea is very flexible because it is less developed. p. 60, Objective 2

18. A. Oxygenated blood is pumped from the lungs into the left atrium, to the left ventricle and then to the body. The average man has approximately 5 L of blood. Platelets are important for blood clotting. White blood cells are important for fighting infection. The upper chambers of the heart are the atria, and the lower chambers are the ventricles. p. 61, Objective 2

19. B. The femur is the thigh. The tibia and fibula are both bones in the lower leg. The patella is the kneecap. p. 66, Objective 2

20. C. The middle layer of the skin is the dermis, the outer layer is the epidermis, and the deeper layer is the subcutaneous level. The central nervous system is composed of the brain and spinal cord. The peripheral nervous system is composed of motor nerves that carry information from the brain to the body and sensory nerves that carry information from the body to the brain. The endocrine system releases hormones in the body. p. 69, Objective 2

21. B. The average pulse rate range for an adult is 60 to 80. These numbers are only the average. A pulse rate higher or lower can be normal for an individual. p. 79, Objective 6

22. D. Bilateral chest expansion means that both lungs are expanding equally. This is associated with normal respirations. Increased effort of breathing, grunting and stridor, and use of accessory muscles all indicate abnormal breathing. p. 80, Objective 4

23. A. The skin temperature can be described as hot, warm, cool, or cold. Dry and clammy are skin conditions; pale is a skin color. p. 82, Objectives 9, 10, 11

24. B. Capillary refill is only assessed in patients less than 6 years of age. Pupils should *constrict* equally when exposed to light. The diastolic pressure is the measurement of force exerted when the heart is at rest. The systolic pressure is the measurement of the forces exerted when the heart is contracting. Vital signs should be assessed every 5 minutes for an unstable patient and every 15 minutes for a stable patient. p. 83, Objectives 14, 18, 20, 21, 25

25. D. The acronym SAMPLE stands for Signs and Symptoms, Allergies, Medications, Past pertinent history, Last oral intake, and Events leading to the illness or injury. A symptom is something the patient must describe to you. A sign is an observable condition. Ask the patient about any allergies, including food, medications, insects, etc. The patient's pertinent past history should be assessed—there is no need for a complete medical history. p. 86, Objective 23

26. A. When lifting, be sure to lift with your legs, not your back. Do not twist your body to move the

patient. Use as many rescuers as necessary to safely lift or move the patient. p. 92, Objective 2

27. C. Do not bend at the waist when lifting. Bending at the waist means that you will be lifting with your back, not your legs. Both the power-lift and power-grip will help the EMT–Basic lift safely. p. 93, Objective 2

28. A. Emergency moves are used when there is immediate danger or when you cannot treat the patient because of the position he/she is in. Spinal protection measures can be taken during urgent moves. A patient with signs and symptoms of shock would require an urgent move. p. 97, Objectives 10, 11

29. A. Unresponsive patients without traumatic injuries should be transported in the recovery position to help maintain an open airway. p. 105, Objective 10

30. D. Responsive patients without traumatic injuries should be transported in the position of comfort. p. 105, Objective 10

● CHAPTER 7
THE AIRWAY

● MATCHING
1. B
2. F
3. S
4. C
5. J
6. H
7. G
8. E
9. D
10. A
11. I
12. M
13. L
14. K
15. O
16. V
17. U
18. R
19. Q
20. W
21. T
22. N
23. X
24. P

Definitions to key terms can be found on page 113 of the student textbook. Key terms cover Objectives 1, 20, and 22.

25. **a.** Nasopharynx; **b.** Oropharynx; **c.** Epiglottis; **d.** Larynx; **e.** Right bronchus; **f.** Diaphragm; **g.** Left bronchus. p. 115, Objective 1

26. **a.** One-way valve; **b.** Self-inflating bag; **c.** Oxygen reservoir valve; **d.** Face mask; **e.** Oxygen supply; **f.** Oxygen reservoir. p. 131, Objective 11

● REVIEW QUESTIONS

1. True. When the diaphragm contracts, it flattens and increases the size of the chest, pulling air into the nose and mouth. p. 114, Objective 2

2. False. Exhalation is normally a passive process, but can be an active process if the patient has respiratory compromise. p. 115, Objective 2

3. C. The normal range of respiratory rates for an adult is 12 to 20 breaths per minute. This is only an average number. A patient may be breathing faster or slower and still be within his/her normal limits. p. 116, Objective 2

4. Signs and symptoms of inadequate breathing include: difficulty breathing or shortness of breath; a rate that is too fast or too slow; an irregular rhythm; diminished or absent breath sounds; unequal or inadequate chest expansion; increased effort of breathing; inadequate tidal volume (shallow breathing); cyanotic, pale, or cool and clammy skin; and use of accessory muscles. Signs of adequate breathing include: adequate rate and depth; regular rhythm; bilateral chest expansion; and no visible labor associated with breathing. p. 117, Objectives 2, 3

5. To deliver oxygen to a patient you will need an oxygen source (such as an oxygen cylinder), a regulator (to get the oxygen at an appropriate rate and pressure), and a delivery device (such as a nonrebreather mask, nasal cannula, or ventilation device). p. 117, Objective 19

6. EMT–Basics commonly use nonrebreather masks and nasal cannulas. EMT–Basics use nonrebreather masks in most cases. If a patient will not tolerate a mask, a nasal cannula may be used. p. 118, Objectives 20, 22

7. C. Nonrebreather masks can deliver up to 90% oxygen when the flow rate is set at 15 L/min. p. 118, Objective 20

8. False. The nasal cannula is a low-flow device and therefore a poor substitute for a nonrebreather mask. The nasal cannula is used only when the patient will not tolerate a mask. p. 120, Objective 21

9. C. The oxygen flow rate can be set up to 6 L/min when using a nasal cannula. p. 120, Objective 22

10. False. The head-tilt, chin-lift is used most commonly to open the airway, unless there is suspected trauma. When there is suspected trauma, the jaw thrust must be used to open the airway. p. 121, Objective 5

11. When performing the head-tilt, chin-lift, with one hand on the forehead, tilt the head back and use the other hand to lift the chin. The jaw thrust is performed by placing your index fingers at the angles of the jaw and the meaty parts of your thumbs on the maxilla, using your thumb tips to keep the mouth open. Both methods are designed to maintain a patent airway. p. 122, Objectives 4, 6

12. Oral airways are measured from the corner of the mouth to the *earlobe* or the *angle of the jaw*. The correct size is important to ensure that the tongue is lifted out of the airway. p. 124, Objective 17

13. B. For infants and children, the preferred method for inserting an oral airway is by using a tongue depressor to lift the tongue out of the airway and then inserting the airway right side up. p. 125, Objective 17

14. True. An oral airway will stimulate the gag reflex of a responsive patient. A nasal airway may be better tolerated. p. 125, Objective 18

15. The nasal airway is measured from the tip of the nose to the *earlobe*. The airway is inserted with the bevel toward the *septum* of the nose. p. 125, Objective 18

16. Gurgling is one of the most common signs of liquid in the airway, and immediate suction is indicated. Suction must be readily available at all times during patient assessment and care. p. 127, Objective 7

17. B. You should only insert the suction catheter as far as you can see. p. 127, Objective 8

18. A. Bulb syringes are used to suction the mouth and nose of infants and children up to 3 or 4 months of age. They must be compressed before being placed into the mouth or nose. p. 127, Objective 8

19. A. Suctioning should not last more than 15 seconds before delivering more oxygen to the patient. p. 129, Objective 8

20. When performing mouth-to-mouth ventilation: open the airway; take a deep breath; pinch the patient's nostrils closed; make a seal with your mouth on the patient's lips; exhale until the chest rises over 1.5 to 2 seconds; and ventilate once every 5 seconds for adults and every 3 seconds for infants and children. p. 140, Objective 16

21. C. Mouth-to-mask is the preferred ventilation technique because it provides excellent ventilatory volumes, requires only one person, allows for a two-hand mask seal, and can be attached to supplemental oxygen. p. 130, Objective 9

22. B. When using the two-person technique, one person maintains the mask seal with both hands and the second squeezes the bag. Two people are preferred when it is difficult for one person to maintain a mask seal. In either technique, ventilate the patient once every 5 seconds for adult patients and once every 3 seconds for infants and children. p. 131, Objective 12

23. D. The flow-restricted, oxygen-powered ventilation device delivers 100% oxygen when the trigger is pushed, at a maximum flow rate of 40 L/min.

The EMT–Basic must maintain an open airway and a good mask seal. This device is not recommended for infants and children because it may cause lung tissue damage and cause air to enter the stomach. p. 132, Objective 15

24. B. The EMT–Basic maintaining the mask seal also can perform the jaw thrust. Do not use the head-tilt, chin-lift for trauma patients. The mask seal is not changed, and the patient should be ventilated once every 5 seconds for adult patients and once every 3 seconds for infants and children. p. 133, Objectives 5, 10

25. Signs of adequate ventilation include: chest rises and falls with each ventilation; heart rate returns to normal; age-appropriate rate; and skin color improves. Signs and symptoms of inadequate ventilation include: failure of the chest to rise and fall with ventilation; rate is too fast or too slow; gastric distention; heart rate does not return to normal; and cyanosis is present or worsens. p. 134, Objectives 13, 14

26. When there is poor chest rise during ventilation: 1) reposition the jaw or head; 2) check the mask seal; 3) try a different technique; and 4) check for an obstruction. p. 134, Objective 10

27. You usually can ventilate a patient with a tracheal stoma with a mask directly through the stoma. Create a seal with the mask, and ventilate as usual using a BVM or mouth-to-mask technique. The head does not need to be positioned, because you are ventilating below the level of the tongue and epiglottis. p. 135, Objective 16

28. False. An oral airway can be used for an unresponsive trauma patient to help maintain an open airway. p. 136, Objective 5

29. True. Dentures and other dental appliances help create a mask seal by giving structure to the face. They should be left in place unless they are so loose that they may cause an obstruction. p. 136

30. a. The airway structures of infants and children are smaller than in adults. The tongue takes up proportionately more space, and the trachea is very narrow and easily obstructed by small amounts of fluid or swelling. p. 116. b. Signs and symptoms of inadequate breathing include: difficulty breathing; shortness of breath; fast or slow rate; irregular rhythm; diminished or absent breath sounds; unequal or inadequate chest expansion; increased breathing effort; inadequate tidal volume; shallow breathing; use of accessory muscles; cyanosis; pallor; and cool, clammy skin. p. 117. c. Tidal volume is the amount of air that a person exchanges in one breath. The easiest way to evaluate tidal volume is to watch the chest rise and fall with each ventilation. If the chest is only moving slightly, tidal volume is inadequate. p. 116

31. a. When ventilating a patient you should observe the chest rise and fall with each ventilation, the heart rate should return to normal, and the skin color should improve. p. 134. b. Other methods of

ventilation include mouth-to-mask ventilation and the flow-restricted, oxygen-powered ventilation device. p. 130. c. The patient's airway may be obstructed causing poor ventilation. You should consider performing the Heimlich maneuver or suctioning the patient's airway. p. 134

● DIVISION TWO EXAMINATION

1. C. The chest expands during inhalation. As the diaphragm contracts and lowers the ribs move upward and outward, increasing the size of the thoracic cavity, so air is pulled into the lungs. p. 114, Objective 1

2. B. The normal respiratory rate in children is between 15 to 30 breaths per minute. It is important to remember that this is only an average range. A child may be breathing faster or slower, and this rate may still be normal for the child. p. 116, Objective 2

3. D. When a patient is breathing adequately, the chest expands equally, there are a normal rate and adequate tidal volume, and breathing is regular and relaxed. Signs and symptoms of inadequate breathing include: difficulty breathing or shortness or breath; a rate that is too fast or too slow; a rhythm that is irregular; diminished or absent breath sounds; unequal or inadequate chest expansion; increased effort of breathing; inadequate tidal volume; cyanotic, pale, or cool and clammy skin; and the use of accessory muscles. p. 117, Objectives 2, 3

4. D. This patient is presenting in respiratory distress with signs and symptoms of poor oxygenation. He needs to receive high-concentration oxygen from a nonrebreather mask. The flow rate should be set at 15 L/min. p. 118, Objectives 20, 21

5. C. The jaw thrust will keep the head in neutral alignment. All of the other techniques listed will move the head, potentially causing damage to the spinal cord. p. 122, Objective 5

6. D. Oral airways may be inserted using a tongue depressor, or you may insert the oral airway upside down until resistance is met, then rotate the airway 180° until the flange rests against the patient's teeth. The oral airway is measured from the corner of the patient's mouth to the angle of the jaw or the earlobe. Oral airways can only be used on patients who do not have a gag reflex. p. 122, Objective 17

7. D. Only insert the suction catheter as far as you can see. For rigid or soft catheters, the suction catheter should never be inserted any further than you can see, usually to about the base of the tongue. p. 127, Objective 8

8. A. If there are large amounts of material in the airway, logroll the patient and clear the airway. After rolling the patient back, suction may be used if necessary. The patient should not be continuously

suctioned without ventilation. You should suction the patient first before you attempt to ventilate to avoid pushing emesis or secretions into the airway. p. 127, Objective 8

9. C. Suction the patient for no longer than 15 seconds before providing oxygen. p. 129, Objective 8

10. The preferred order for ventilation devices for EMT–Basics set forth in the National Standard Curriculum are: 1) Mouth-to-mask; 2) Two-person, bag-valve-mask; 3) Flow-restricted, oxygen-powered ventilation device; and 4) One-person, bag-valve-mask. p. 129

11. B. Bag-valve-masks should not have pop-off valves. Pop-off valves may lead to ventilating with too little air. The bag-valve-mask should have a self-refilling bag that is either disposable or easily cleaned and sterilized, an oxygen inlet and standardized fittings, and a one-way valve, and should work in all temperatures and come in a variety of sizes. p. 132, Objective 11

12. C. When ventilating using a flow-restricted, oxygen-powered ventilation device, the alarm should sound when the relief valve pressure exceeds 60 cm of water. Flow-restricted, oxygen-powered ventilation devices can deliver up to 100% oxygen at a peak flow rate of 40 L/min. The device allows the EMT–Basic to use both hands to ventilate the patient. p. 132, Objective 15

13. A. The neck and head must remain in the neutral position, so the head and neck are stabilized before ventilation. Any procedure that tilts the head should not be used when there is suspected cervical spine trauma. The ventilation rate of once every 5 seconds for adults and once every 3 seconds for infants and children does not change for trauma patients. p. 133, Objective 5

14. B. EMT–Basics need to avoid excessive bag pressure when ventilating an infant or child, because gastric distention is more likely and causes problems when ventilating. Pop-off valves should not be used because ventilation may occur with too little volume. The head should be in a neutral position for infants and tilted slightly further back for children, avoiding kinking the trachea. p. 136, Objective 12

15. B. If dentures or other dental appliances become dislodged, they may become an airway obstruction and should be removed. p. 137

● **CHAPTER 8**
SCENE SIZE-UP

● **MATCHING**
1. C
2. A
3. B

Definitions to key terms can be found on page 143 of the student textbook.

● **REVIEW QUESTIONS**

1. True. Personal protection includes body substance isolation precautions to prevent exposure to blood and other body fluids and protective clothing such as turnout gear and helmets. Personal protective equipment will vary with each situation. p. 145, Objective 3

2. C. Patient assessment does not occur during the scene size-up. The scene size-up occurs before you enter the scene and is designed to protect you and your crew from injury and to help identify any need for additional resources. p. 145, Objective 3

3. Many hazards may be present at an automobile crash. Some of these hazards include: broken glass, torn metal, gasoline, angry bystanders, and traffic hazards. Each scene has its own potential hazards, so keep alert and look for danger. p. 145, Objectives 1, 2

4. Although hazards at the scene of a medical call are not as common or obvious as at the scene of a trauma call, the EMT–Basic still must be alert and look for hazards. Hazards may include people (for example, a violent person on scene or a mentally unstable patient), animals (a protective dog), the environment (such as extreme heat or cold, or carbon monoxide or natural gas in the air), and exposure to blood or other body fluids. p. 145, Objective 2

5. You must use your senses to evaluate the scene and determine if there are any hazards. Look at, listen to, and smell the environment to determine if there are any unsafe situations or substances present. p. 145, Objective 3

6. If the scene is not safe and you can not make it safe, do not enter the scene. EMT–Basics will not be able to help the patient if they are injured themselves. p. 145

7. A. The nature of illness is also called the chief complaint. The chief complaint usually describes the reason why EMS was called. p. 147, Objective 4

8. True. You can usually determine many of the factors of the mechanism of injury by observing the patient's surroundings, but you cannot always discover every factor that may have caused injury to the patient. p. 147, Objective 4

9. Identifying the mechanism of injury will help you determine if there are any hidden internal injuries, in addition to the external ones you can see. p. 148, Objective 4

10. Taking time to determine the total number of patients at the scene early in the scene size-up will allow you to request additional resources if there are more patients than the personnel on scene can handle. While determining the number of patients,

age- or gender-specific articles, such as a baby car seat or a woman's purse, may indicate the presence of an unseen patient. p. 148, Objective 5

11. The scene size-up will help you determine if additional help is necessary. Additional help should be requested for lifting assistance for a large patient, to control traffic, to deal with hazardous materials, for fire suppression or electrical lines, to provide rescue equipment, or if there are too many patients for the available personnel to handle. p. 148, Objective 6

12. **a.** Consider the need for body substance isolation precautions and don protective gear. Because shots have been fired, there is a potential for contact with blood and other body fluids. p. 145. **b.** Ensure your own safety before addressing the safety of the patient or bystanders. Once you are sure the scene is safe, proceed with patient care. p. 145. **c.** The scene has become unsafe, and you should move to a safe area. p. 145

13. **a.** During the scene size-up, you should check for scene safety, determine the mechanism of injury, determine how may patients are involved, and evaluate the need for additional help. p. 145. **b.** Look for the presence of broken glass, torn metal, hazardous fluids, and bystanders. Notice if there are any unusual odors (*eg*, gasoline). Listen for expected and unexpected sounds (*eg*, an engine running, arcing wires). p. 145. **c.** Protect the patient from metal, flying glass, or sparks created by extrication tools. Provide protection from the environment, such as extreme heat or cold. p. 146

● CHAPTER 9
INITIAL ASSESSMENT

● REVIEW QUESTIONS

1. EMT–Basics form a general impression to determine the patient's priority of care and to form a plan of action for continuing to assess the patient and provide care. p. 154, Objective 1

2. B. The general impression is formed in seconds by simply looking at and listening to your patient. The patient's name is not necessary to form your general impression, although you may ask the patient his/her name early in your interaction to establish rapport. While forming a general impression, determine the nature of illness or mechanism of injury; the patient's age, race and gender; and if there are any life-threatening injuries. p. 155, Objective 1

3. False. You will need to assess the mental status of a child in different ways based on the child's age. Older children should be able to answer simple questions. Young children may only be able to tell

you their name. Children of all ages prefer to be with their parents rather than strangers. A child who does not respond when removed from the parents is not alert. Children will try to locate their parents' voices or will be startled by loud verbal stimuli. Assess response to pain in the same manner as you would an adult, with a mildly painful stimulus. p. 156, Objective 3

4. An alert patient will talk to you without prompting. If a patient is not alert, talk to the patient to determine if he/she is responsive to verbal stimuli. If the patient does not respond, test if there is response to a painful stimulus. A painful stimulus should be strong enough to cause a reaction from the patient, but not strong enough to injure the patient. A pinch on the shoulder, the fingers, or the foot is sufficient to elicit a painful response. If the patient does not respond to painful stimuli, he/she is unresponsive. p. 156, Objective 2

5. False. Mental status changes are one of the most sensitive indicators of changes in the patient's condition. Patients often become restless or confused very early when they are becoming hypoxic or going into shock. p. 156, Objective 2

6. C. The head-tilt, chin-lift is the most common way to open the airway of a medical patient. The head-tilt, chin-lift will cause a change in the alignment of the spine and should not be used for trauma patients. The jaw thrust should be used for trauma patients because the head will remain in the neutral position. p. 157, Objective 4

7. The head of a trauma patient is stabilized in the neutral position to prevent any movement of the head, which will, in turn, move the spine. It is important to minimize movements of the spine to protect the patient from further injury. The jaw thrust is used for trauma patients because the head-tilt, chin-lift also will move the spine. p. 157, Objective 5

8. EMT–Basics should administer oxygen to an adult patient breathing less than *eight* times per minute or greater than *24* times per minute. If the patient is breathing adequately, but is unresponsive, help maintain a(n) *open or patent* airway and administer *high-flow* oxygen. If a patient is breathing adequately, the EMT–Basic should follow local protocol regarding administration of oxygen to the patient. If the patient is breathing inadequately, apply oxygen via a nonrebreather mask or by assisting the patient's ventilations with a BVM, mouth-to-mask, or flow-restricted, oxygen-powered ventilation device. p. 157, Objectives 7, 8, 9

9. You can determine if a patient is breathing by opening the airway and watching the rise and fall of the chest. You would assess the respiratory efforts by checking the rate and quality. p. 157, Objective 6

10. False. EMT–Basics should assess the rate and quality of breathing of an infant or child the same way as for an adult. The normal range of respiratory rates of infants and children is higher than for adults but still should be evaluated. A slow respiratory rate for an infant or child can be a sign of a serious respiratory problem. Care for infants and children is the same as for an adult. p. 158, Objectives 10, 11

11. False. Life-threatening conditions should be cared for as they are found. Do not wait to begin to correct a life-threatening condition such as an airway obstruction or major bleeding. p. 157, Objective 1

12. A. Initially assess the adult or child patient's pulse by palpating the radial artery. If the radial pulse cannot be felt, palpate the carotid pulse. For infants, begin by assessing the brachial pulse. p. 158, Objectives 12, 13

13. The EMT–Basic first assesses for external bleeding during the *general impression* and again when evaluating the patient's *circulation*. You may need to remove clothing from a trauma patient to properly evaluate for external bleeding. Any major bleeding should be considered a life threat and should be controlled immediately. p. 158, Objective 14

14. Normal skin color is pink when evaluated at the nail beds, inside of the lips or inside the eyelids. Abnormal skin colors include pale (poor perfusion), cyanotic (inadequate oxygenation), flushed (hot or exposed to carbon monoxide), or jaundiced (poor liver function). The skin is normally warm. Abnormal skin temperatures include hot (exposure to heat or fever), cool (exposure to cold or poor perfusion), cold (exposure to extreme cold), or clammy (cold and moist, sign of hypoperfusion). The skin condition is normally dry. Abnormal skin conditions include moist (possible sign of shock), wet (possible sign of shock), and extremely dry (dehydration). p. 159, Objectives 15, 16, 17

15. False. Capillary refill should take less than 2 seconds to return to normal. Assess capillary refill by pushing on the nail bed until it blanches and then count the time it takes for the color to return to normal. Assess capillary refill on patients younger than 6 years of age. p. 159, Objective 18

16. B. Patients with severe pain anywhere are considered to be priority patients. Other priority patients include any patient who: has a poor general impression; is unresponsive with no gag reflex or cough; is responsive but unable to follow commands; has difficulty breathing; has signs and symptoms of shock; has complicated childbirth; has chest pain and a blood pressure of less than 100 systolic; and has uncontrolled bleeding. p. 160, Objective 19

17. During the initial assessment, determine the patient's priority for care so that priority patients can be rapidly transported to the receiving facility.

Time should not be wasted on scene with further assessment of these patients. All further assessments can take place in the back of the ambulance en route to the closest appropriate receiving facility. p. 160, Objective 19

18. **a.** During the initial assessment, form a general impression; assess mental status; assess the airway; assess breathing, rate, and quality; assess circulation; identify any life-threatening injuries and provide appropriate care; and make an initial decision. p. 154. **b.** Initiate spinal precautions, position the patient, and open his airway. The blood, vomit, and teeth must be cleared before performing any other assessments or care. p. 155. **c.** Using the AVPU categories, the patient is "P" (painful) because he responds only to painful stimulus. p. 156

19. **a.** The 27-year-old patient shot in the chest has a potential for displaying the signs and symptoms of shock. p. 160. **b.** Contact dispatch and request ALS intercept or ALS back-up; notify dispatch to send additional crew members to the scene. p. 160. **c.** Priority patients who: have poor general impression; are unresponsive with no gag reflex or cough; are responsive but unable to follow commands; have difficulty breathing; have signs and symptoms of shock; have complicated childbirth; have chest pain and a blood pressure less than 100 systolic; have uncontrolled bleeding; and have severe pain anywhere. p. 160

● CHAPTER 10
FOCUSED HISTORY AND PHYSICAL EXAMINATION FOR TRAUMA PATIENTS

● MATCHING

1. C
2. G
3. E
4. F
5. H
6. B
7. A
8. I
9. D

Definitions to key terms can be found on page 165 of the student textbook.

● REVIEW QUESTIONS

1. The mechanism of injury will help guide the EMT–Basic toward the patient's injuries. A serious mechanism of injury will help the EMT–Basic to search for hidden injuries or maintain a high index of suspicion when a patient appears to be only slightly injured. p. 167, Objective 1

2. B. Falls are considered to be a high-risk mechanism of injury when the height is greater than 20 feet. Other significant mechanisms of injury include: the ejection of driver or passenger from a vehicle; being in a car where another person died; vehicle roll-over; high-speed vehicle collision; vehicle-pedestrian collision; motorcycle crash; patients who are unresponsive or who have an altered mental status; and penetrating trauma to the head, chest, or abdomen. p. 167, Objective 1

3. True. Older patients and very young patients are more easily injured than healthy adults. A less serious mechanism of injury may result in a serious injury to these patients. p. 167, Objective 2

4. D—Deformities; C—Contusions; A—Abrasions; P—Penetrations; B—Burns; T—Tenderness; L—Lacerations; S—Swelling. p. 168, Objective 4

5. The rapid trauma assessment should take approximately *60 to 90* seconds. With practice, you should be able to complete the rapid trauma assessment in less than 90 seconds. p. 168, Objective 2

6. Anytime a life-threatening condition is discovered, the assessment should be stopped long enough to care for the condition and then you should continue the assessment. p. 168, Objective 5

7. B. Auscultate the bases of the lungs at the midaxillary line and the apices at the midclavicular line to determine if breath sounds are present and equal. p. 170, Objective 4

8. A. Most patients will have a soft abdomen at rest. A firm or rigid abdomen can be a sign of injury to the abdomen or blood accumulating in the abdomen. When palpating the abdomen, gently push against all four quadrants, feeling for rigidity and noticing if the palpation causes the patient any pain. p. 170, Objective 4

9. C. When evaluating the pelvis, flex the pelvis by pushing posteriorly on the iliac wings and then compress by pushing toward the midline. Do not assess the pelvis if the patient has any pain in the pelvic region or if the mechanism of injury suggests that the patient may have injured the pelvis. If the pelvis is painful or unstable during the first examination of the pelvis, do not repeat this step of the examination. p. 170, Objective 4

10. When evaluating the extremities, assess for DCAP-BTLS and distal pulse, motor function, and sensation. Ask patients if they can feel you touching their extremity and if they can move their fingers and toes slightly. p. 171, Objective 4

11. False. If the patient has a serious mechanism of injury, you should perform the rapid trauma assessment, even if the patient only complains of an isolated injury. Patients often are not aware of their most serious injury, only the most painful injury. p. 173, Objective 3

12. False. Not every patient will require a rapid trauma assessment. If the patient has no serious mechanism of injury and complains only of an isolated injury, you can direct your assessment toward the injury. A patient who dropped a heavy object on his/her foot will not require a head-to-toe trauma assessment. p. 173, Objective 3

13. False. Patients often only are aware of the most painful injury, not necessarily the most serious. The mechanism of injury and the information obtained during the rest of the focused history and physical examination will help you determine if the patient should receive a rapid trauma assessment. p. 173, Objective 6

14. F. This is an isolated injury with no serious mechanism of injury. p. 173, Objective 3

15. F. This patient has an isolated injury to her ankle and no serious mechanism of injury. p. 173, Objective 3

16. R. This patient has sustained a serious mechanism of injury. Even though he appears to be uninjured, a trauma assessment is needed. p. 173, Objective 3

17. **a.** Yes. Falls of greater than 20 feet are considered to be high risk for hidden injury. p. 167. **b.** Because the patient is responsive you could obtain a SAMPLE history, including the cause of the event, during the initial assessment. This would include the reason for the fall (*eg*, loss of balance) and whether there was an associated loss of responsiveness before or after the fall. You also could ask the patient to describe any pain or discomfort that resulted from the fall. p. 168. **c.** A patient who has sustained a significant mechanism of injury should be prepared for transport with full spinal precautions. p. 169

18. **a.** Your first priority is to secure the patient's airway. This includes positioning the patient and opening her airway while maintaining spinal precautions. Suction the airway as needed. p. 168. **b.** Before beginning the assessment, control the airway and manually stabilize the head and spine. p. 168. **c.** You would assess this patient for deformities, contusions, abrasions, penetrations or punctures, burns, tenderness, lacerations, and swelling. Based on the mechanism of injury, this patient may have sustained trauma to every body system, so the rapid trauma assessment is indicated. p. 168

● CHAPTER 11
FOCUSED HISTORY AND PHYSICAL EXAMINATION FOR MEDICAL PATIENTS

● MATCHING

1. A
2. C

3. B

4. D

Definitions to key terms can be found on page 177 of the student textbook.

● REVIEW QUESTIONS

1. False. A responsive medical patient receives a focused history and physical examination based on the chief complaint. An unresponsive medical patient receives the rapid trauma assessment to evaluate for trauma and to complete a head-to-toe assessment. p. 179, Objectives 2, 3

2. O—Onset; P—Provocation; Q—Quality; R—Radiation; S—Severity; T—Time. p. 179, Objective 4

3. P—What position makes you feel better? Provocation or palliation means "what makes the pain worse or better?" p. 179, Objective 4

4. O—How long have you had cardiac problems? Onset refers to the beginning of the patient's condition. p. 179, Objective 4

5. T—How long have you had this pain? Time refers to the time when this specific episode began. p. 179, Objective 4

6. S—Is this the worst pain you've ever had? Severity is often scored on a scale from 1 to 10, with 10 being the worst pain the patient ever felt. p. 179, Objective 4

7. P—What makes the pain worse? Provocation is what makes the pain worse. p. 179, Objective 4

8. R—Does the pain spread or move? Radiation refers to any movement of the pain. p. 179, Objective 4

9. Q—Can you describe the pain you are feeling? Quality of pain is how the patient describes the feeling. Let the patient describe the pain in his/her own words. p. 179, Objective 4

10. True. EMT–Basics should always ask patients information regarding their history. Valuable information can be gained and forwarded to the referring facility. p. 180, Objective 4

11. S—signs and symptoms; A—allergies; M—current medications; P—past medical history; L—last food or drink; E—events leading to this illness. p. 180, Objective 4

12. The focused history and physical examination for the medical patient is guided by the patient's *chief complaint*. There is generally no reason for the EMT–Basic to perform a head-to-toe assessment on a responsive medical patient with no history of trauma. p. 180, Objective 1

13. If the patient has a known medical condition, there may be a change in the way the EMT–Basic cares for that patient. For example, if the patient has a history of cardiac disease, the patient's physician may have prescribed the medication nitroglycerin.

If the patient has nitroglycerin, in some instances the EMT–Basic can assist the patient with administration of the medication. p. 182, Objectives 1, 2

14. True. To help determine what may be wrong with the unresponsive medical patient, EMT–Basics should perform a focused history and physical examination as they would for the trauma patient. A head-to-toe rapid trauma assessment should be performed. p. 182, Objective 3

15. When a medical patient is unresponsive and cannot provide a SAMPLE history, information can be obtained from *family members or bystanders*. If no family members are present, ask bystanders to describe what they witnessed. p. 183, Objective 3

16. C. Place unresponsive medical patients with no history of trauma in the recovery position to help maintain a patent airway. p. 183, Objective 3

17. **a.** The "O" signifies onset or origin of the patient's medical problem. Questions to ask this patient include "Do you have a history of cardiac diseases?" and "How long have you had a cardiac condition?" p. 179. **b.** The "Q" signifies the quality of the pain. Questions to ask this patient include "Can you describe the discomfort you are feeling?" p. 180. **c.** The "T" signifies duration of time since the patient felt it necessary to call EMS. Questions to ask include "How long have you been experiencing this chest discomfort?" and "What happened to make you call EMS?" p. 180

18. **a.** After ensuring scene safety, assessment and control of the airway with spinal precautions is your first priority. p. 183. **b.** Because the patient is unresponsive and cannot direct you toward her illness or injury, the focused history and physical examination for a trauma patient would be indicated. You would perform a rapid trauma assessment on this patient. p. 183. **c.** If you can be certain there was no trauma involved, transport the patient in the recovery position to allow secretions to drain from her mouth and to help maintain an open airway. Otherwise, immobilize the patient to a long spine board. p. 183

● CHAPTER 12
DETAILED PHYSICAL EXAMINATION

● REVIEW QUESTIONS

1. True. The rapid trauma assessment is generally performed quickly on scene (within 60 to 90 seconds), where lighting may or may not be ideal. The detailed physical examination is slower and occurs in the back of the ambulance, where the lighting may be better. p. 188, Objective 1

2. False. Not every trauma patient will receive a detailed physical examination. Patients with iso-

lated trauma and no significant mechanism of injury will not require a detailed physical examination. Some trauma patients may be so severely injured that the EMT–Basics spend all of their time evaluating and managing airway, breathing, and circulation and never have time to complete a detailed physical examination. p. 188, Objective 1

3. True. This patient was involved in a crash with serious mechanism of injury and should receive a detailed physical examination. p. 188, Objective 1

4. EMT–Basics will perform a detailed physical examination for medical patients who are unresponsive. Because the patient cannot direct you toward a specific chief complaint, a head-to-toe examination may help you determine the cause of the unresponsiveness or to help you determine if the patient has any traumatic injuries. For medical patients with a specific chief complaint, examining the specific involved body area may be all that is necessary. p. 188, Objective 4

5. Fill in the blanks with the appropriate terms: D—Deformities; C—Contusions; A—Abrasions; P—Penetrations; B—Burns; T—Tenderness; L—Lacerations; S—Swelling. p. 189, Objective 2

6. False. When evaluating the ears, nose, and mouth during the detailed physical examination, use a penlight to look for drainage or trauma. During the rapid trauma assessment, the ears, nose, and mouth are examined quickly. Performing the detailed physical examination gives you the opportunity to carefully examine these areas. p. 189, Objective 2

7. When evaluating the neck, you should assess for DCAP-BTLS and jugular vein distension (JVD). If the cervical spine immobilization device has already been applied, it may need to be removed for this examination. p. 190, Objective 2

8. The patient's pelvis should be examined unless he/she has complaints of pain or if the mechanism of injury suggests a pelvic injury. Do not reevaluate the patient's pelvis if it was unstable or painful during the first assessment. In all other cases, the pelvis should be evaluated by flexing and compressing the pelvic girdle to determine stability. p. 191, Objective 2

9. C. The detailed assessment should, ideally, be performed in the back of the ambulance, en route to the receiving facility. If there is no means of transporting the patient, the detailed physical examination can be performed on scene. p. 192, Objective 2

10. a. Yes. All patients with a significant mechanism of injury should receive a detailed physical examination. p. 189. b. DCAP-BTLS. Deformities, contusions, abrasions, penetrations/punctures, burns, tenderness, lacerations, swelling. p. 189. c. Because of the fall, you would suspect a possible spine injury. Have your partner manually stabilize the patient's neck for DCAP-BTLS, jugular vein disten-

sion, and crepitation. Then, apply a cervical spine immobilization device and secure the patient to a long backboard. p. 190

11. a. No. The detailed physical examination is indicated for trauma patients and unresponsive patients who may have hidden injuries that are not revealed in the initial assessment. Your initial assessment of this patient identified the nature of his injury. p. 188. b. Assessment of the injury would be limited to DCAP-BTLS on the injured body surface. p. 189. c. Yes. The patient's condition allows for assessment of blood pressure, pulse, and respirations. p. 192

● CHAPTER 13
ONGOING ASSESSMENT

● REVIEW QUESTIONS

1. The ongoing assessment allows the EMT–Basic to reevaluate the patient's condition, to check the accuracy of the interventions, and to document trends in the patient's condition. Trends or changes in the patient's condition can provide valuable clues to the receiving facility about the patient's status and can help them make decisions about their care. p. 198, Objectives 1, 3

2. The initial assessment includes: checking the mental status; evaluating the airway patency; assessing breathing rate and quality; assessing pulse rate and quality; assessing skin color, temperature, condition, and perfusion; and reestablishing patient priority. p. 199, Objective 1

3. Stable patients are reassessed every 15 minutes. Unstable patients are reassessed every 5 minutes. Anytime a patient's condition changes, be sure to reevaluate the patient, and change the status to unstable if appropriate. p. 198, Objective 2

4. Number the following steps in the ongoing assessment: 5—assess skin color, temperature, condition, perfusion; 1—assess mental status; 4—assess pulse; 2—assess airway patency; 3—assess breathing rate and quality; 6—reassess patient priority. p. 199, Objective 2

5. False. The EMT–Basic should reevaluate the patient's chief complaint during the ongoing assessment. Although chief complaints do not usually change, the patient may be more descriptive about the illness or injury. p. 200, Objective 2

6. An isolated set of vital signs does not provide the EMT–Basic with much information. Successive sets of vital signs show changes in the patient's condition over time and allow the EMT–Basic to establish a baseline for the patient. Comparing successive sets of vital signs over time is called trending. p. 200, Objective 3

7. The EMT–Basic should check any intervention that was performed to make sure it is still functioning properly. Examples of interventions to check include: the oxygen supply and delivery system; the adequacy of artificial ventilations; dressings are still controlling bleeding; splints are still immobilizing extremities without being too tight; and straps on the backboard are still immobilizing the patient. If any of the interventions is inadequate, it should be corrected immediately. p. 201, Objective 2

8. **a.** This patient is unstable. The ongoing assessment should be repeated every 5 minutes or less. p. 198. **b.** You should interact constantly with the patient throughout transport. This allows you to observe the patient's mental status and to note any changes for either better or worse. p. 199. **c.** If the patient is unresponsive, check the response to verbal and painful stimuli to establish mental status. p. 199

9. **a.** Check to ensure the flow rate is set at 15 L/min. p. 201. **b.** Ensure that oxygen is adequately flowing; the mask is a nonrebreather; the reservoir bag remains inflated; and enough oxygen remains in the cylinder for the duration of the trip. p. 201. **c.** If the patient cannot be convinced to keep a nonrebreather mask in place, apply a nasal cannula; ensure that the prongs are placed correctly in the patient's nose; set the rate at 6 L/min; and ensure that the oxygen is flowing adequately. The nasal cannula is a low-flow device, which delivers low concentrations of oxygen, and is a poor substitute for the nonrebreather mask. p. 201

● CHAPTER 14
COMMUNICATIONS

● MATCHING
1. C
2. A
3. B
4. D

Definitions to key terms can be found on page 205 of the student textbook.

● REVIEW QUESTIONS
1. B. A base station is a radio at a stationary site with superior transmission and receiving capabilities. A repeater is a remote receiver that receives a transmission from a low-power radio and transmits at a higher power. An encoder is part of a digital system that blocks out radio transmissions not intended for certain units. p. 207, Objective 1

2. The agency that regulates and monitors radio transmissions is called the Federal Communications Commission (FCC). p. 208, Objective 1

3. Monitor the frequency for 5 seconds before transmitting to ensure that the frequency is clear. Transmitting without monitoring the frequency may result in interruptions of other medical care professionals. p. 208, Objective 1

4. C. Wait for 1 second after pushing the push-to-talk button to ensure that your entire transmission is heard. p. 208, Objective 1

5. The phrase *stand-by* means you should wait until you are given a go-ahead to begin transmitting. p. 209, Objective 1

6. True. Everyday language will reduce confusion in radio communications. p. 209, Objective 3

7. False. Courtesy is always assumed. Continuously saying "please" and "thank you" takes up valuable time on the radio. p. 209, Objective 3

8. C. It is not necessary to communicate with dispatch when you are loading the patient. Communicate with dispatch when you receive the call, respond to the call, arrive at the scene, arrive at the patient's side, leave the scene for the receiving facility, arrive at the receiving facility, leave the hospital for the station, and arrive at the station. p. 210, Objective 9

9. B. The radio report should be concise, organized, and pertinent. Avoid lengthy or comprehensive reports over the radio. A longer and more detailed report can be given at bedside. All of the pertinent information that the receiving hospital will require is also documented in the written report. p. 210, Objectives 3, 4

10. The standard medical reporting format includes patient's age and gender; chief complaint; history of present illness; pertinent past medical history; mental status; assessment findings; vital signs; emergency care given; response to emergency care; estimated time to load the patient for transport; estimated travel time from the scene to the hospital; and opportunity for questions from the receiving facility or medical direction physician. p. 210, Objectives 2, 4

11. Tips for effective communication include: verbalize your support; be a good listener; offer a reassuring touch; be respectful; separate personal bias; and be silent when appropriate. Good communicators will evaluate the situation and communicate with the patient and family members based on the situation. p. 212, Objectives 5, 7, 8

12. True. Body language is communicated without words, by such things as posture, facial expression, and tone of voice. p. 212, Objective 8

13. **a.** The standard medical reporting format includes: the patient's age and gender; chief complaint; history of present illness; pertinent past history; mental status; assessment findings; vital signs; emergency care given; response to emergency care; estimated time to load the patient for transport;

and estimated travel time to the hospital. p. 210. **b.** Allow an opportunity for questions from the receiving facility or medical direction physician before ending your report. p. 210. **c.** Any time you are unclear about an order, ask questions that will help clarify the physician's order. p. 210

14. **a.** Use a calm, reassuring voice and age-appropriate language. Be sure to explain everything you are doing and be honest. p. 212. **b.** Do not assume that elderly patients cannot hear you; introduce yourself and assess their ability to hear you; consider how fast you are speaking; slow down and allow the patient to process your questions; use simple terms. p. 212. **c.** Use an interpreter; write notes; be patient; do not show signs of frustration. p. 212

● CHAPTER 15
DOCUMENTATION

● MATCHING

1. D
2. A
3. E
4. B
5. F
6. C

Definitions to key terms can be found on page 217 of the student textbook.

● REVIEW QUESTIONS

1. True. Trending means comparing *trends* in a patient's condition over time, by comparing sets of information. p. 218

2. D. The time of arrival is part of the administrative information set. All of the other elements are part of the patient care data set. p. 219, Objective 1

3. 1 am—*0100*; 6:30 pm—*1830*; 12 noon—*1200*; 4:20 am—*0420*; 10:30 pm—*2230*; 8:25 pm—*2025*; 2:40 am—*0240*; 12:30 am—*0030*. p. 220, Objective 3

4. True. The prehospital care report is used to document what care the EMT–Basic provided for the patient. This document is also a legal record of events at the scene and care provided. EMT–Basics must be careful to document all events that happened at the scene and to be truthful when documenting care given. p. 220, Objective 5

5. O—I saw him drinking at that bar; S—The patient was drunk; S—It looked like the car was going over the speed limit; O—Her blood pressure was 120/80 and the pulse was 72; O—The patient's skin is cool, clammy, and moist to the touch; p. 220, Objective 3

6. The primary function of the prehospital care report is to document care given to the patient.

The prehospital care report also is used as an educational tool, for billing purposes, for research, for evaluation, and for continuous quality improvement. p. 223, Objective 5

7. Most prehospital care report forms have a section for writing a patient *narrative*, allowing EMT–Basics to write about the events in the standard medical reporting format. The narrative should describe facts and record observations in an objective manner. p. 223, Objectives 2, 3

8. Chief complaint—CC; gun shotwound—GSW; every—q; shortness of breath—SOB; history—Hx; immediately—stat; treatment—Rx; alcohol—EtOH. p. 224, Objective 3

9. False. Errors should be corrected by drawing a single line through the error, initialing beside the error, and then writing in the correct information. p. 226, Objectives 3, 5

10. Refusal is the right of any *competent* adult. Patients must be informed about their decisions and able to make a rational decision. p. 227, Objective 4

11. Special situation reports should be used when there is an infectious disease exposure, injury to the EMT–Basic or bystanders, equipment damage or malfunction, vehicle crashes involving the response unit, patient refusals, abuse or neglect, crime scenes, and hazardous materials incidents. Individual EMS systems may have additional special reports used in their region or state. p. 228, Objective 6

12. **a.** Patient information and administrative information are both part of the minimum data set. p. 219. **b.** Pertinent information includes: age and gender; chief complaint; cause of injury; preexisting conditions; signs and symptoms present; injury description; level of responsiveness (AVPU); pulse rate; respiratory rate; systolic blood pressure in patients over 3 years of age; skin perfusion; skin color, temperature, and condition; procedures performed on the patient; medications administered; and response to treatment, including medications. p. 219. **c.** For administrative purposes, gather the following information: incident location; type of location; date and time the incident was reported; date and time the EMS unit was notified; time the unit responded; time of arrival at the scene; time of arrival at the patient; time EMS left the scene; time EMS arrived at destination; time of transfer of patient care; time the EMS unit was back in service; use of lights and sirens; and crew members responding. p. 219

13. **a.** Yes. All competent adults have the right to refuse treatment for themselves or others in their care. p. 227. **b.** Inform the patient why treatment and transport are necessary and what may happen without treatment; contact medical direction; and have a physician speak with the patient. p. 227.

c. Document your assessment findings; have the patient sign a refusal form; document that you have informed the patient of adverse effects that may result from not accepting care or transportation, including possible death; have a family member, police officer, or bystander sign the form as a witness; before leaving the scene, tell the patient about other ways to receive care; and state and document your willingness to return for treatment and transportation. p. 228

● DIVISION THREE EXAMINATION

1. B. BSI precautions are designed to protect the EMT–Basic from blood-borne and air-borne pathogens. Need for BSI precautions should be determined in the scene size-up. BSI precautions should be used anytime there is a chance of contact with any body fluid, not just blood. p. 145, Objective 1

2. B. The EMT–Basic should always be concerned with his/her own safety first. If the EMT–Basic is injured, he/she will not be able to help anyone at the scene. After personal safety, priorities include safety of other crew members, patient safety, and bystander safety. p. 145, Objective 3

3. A. During the scene size-up, the EMT–Basic will determine scene safety, the mechanism of injury or nature of illness, the number of patients, and the need for additional help. No patient information will be obtained during the scene size-up. p. 145, Objective 3

4. A. During the scene size-up, EMT–Basics should check for scene safety, determine the nature of illness or mechanism of injury, determine the number of patients present, and call for additional help if necessary. If there are too many patients for the EMT–Basics on scene to treat, call for additional help and begin treating the most seriously injured patients. No patient care takes place during the scene size-up. p. 149, Objectives 5, 6

5. C. During the general impression, the EMT–Basic determines the patient's age, gender, and race; mechanism of injury or nature of illness; and if any life threats are present. Form a general impression in the first few seconds, before any additional patient assessment is performed. p. 154, Objective 1

6. B. The AVPU acronym stands for Alert, responsive to Verbal stimuli, responsive to Painful stimuli, or Unresponsive. AVPU is used to categorize a patient's mental status. p. 155, Objective 2

7. C. A slow respiratory rate is a threat to life and should be treated immediately. Have your partner ventilate the patient using a pocket mask, one- or two-person bag-valve-mask, or a flow-restricted, oxygen-powered ventilation device. p. 157, Objective 8

8. B. For alert adult patients, assess the radial pulse first. If the adult or child patient is unresponsive or if you cannot feel a radial pulse, evaluate the carotid pulse. Evaluate the brachial pulse for infants. p. 158, Objective 13

9. A. To assess perfusion, the EMT–Basic should look at the skin color of the nail beds, the inside of the lips, or the inside the eyelids. The normal skin color in these areas is pink, regardless of race. p. 159, Objective 15

10. D. If the radial pulse is weaker than the carotid pulse, this may be a sign of hypoperfusion. Skin color should be assessed at the nail beds, inside the lips, or inside the eyelids. Temperature should be assessed on the trunk, not the extremities. Capillary refill is an accurate measure of perfusion for children younger than 6 years of age. p. 159, Objectives 15, 16

11. A. A patient who is unresponsive with no gag reflex is a priority patient. Other priority patients include patients: who have poor general impression; who are responsive but unable to follow commands; who are experiencing difficulty breathing; who have signs and symptoms of shock; who are having complicated childbirth; who have chest pain and a blood pressure of less than 100 systolic; who have uncontrolled bleeding; and who have severe pain anywhere. p. 160, Objective 19

12. A. If the patient is involved in a crash where another occupant in the same vehicle compartment died, the patient may have sustained a significant mechanism of injury. Other significant mechanisms of injury include: ejection of driver or passenger from a vehicle; a fall of more than 6 m (20 ft); vehicle roll-over; high-speed vehicle collision; vehicle-pedestrian collision; motorcycle crash; unresponsive patients or patients with an altered mental status; and patients with penetrating trauma to the head, chest, or abdomen. p. 167, Objective 1

13. C. The rapid trauma assessment should take 60 to 90 seconds for most patients. EMT–Basics will be able to perform the trauma assessment rapidly with practice. p. 168, Objective 4

14. A. The acronym DCAP-BTLS stands for Deformities, Contusions, Abrasions, Penetrations, Burns, Tenderness, Lacerations, and Swelling. p. 168, Objective 4

15. C. The abdomen should be evaluated for DCAP-BTLS and softness, tenderness, and distention. p. 171, Objective 4

16. C. If the patient has an isolated injury and no serious mechanism of injury, the EMT–Basic may choose to evaluate the isolated injury only. If there is any doubt about the seriousness of the injury, a complete rapid trauma assessment should be performed. p. 173, Objective 3

17. C. The acronym OPQRST is used to remember what questions to ask during the focused history and physical examination for medical patients when evaluating their chief complaint. The acronym stands for Onset, Provocation, Quality, Radiation, Severity, and Time. p. 179, Objective 1

18. A. Emergency care for patients is based on the assessment findings of the focused history and physical examination and advice from medical direction. Unresponsive medical patients are treated much like unresponsive trauma patients. Unresponsive medical patients with no suspected trauma should be placed in the recovery position. All patients receive an initial assessment, including an evaluation of their airway, breathing, and circulation. p. 180, Objective 3

19. A. The "S" in the SAMPLE history stands for Signs and Symptoms, the "A" for Allergies, the "M" for Medications, the "P" for Past pertinent history, the "L" for Last oral intake, and the "E" for Events leading to the illness or injury. p. 180, Objective 2

20. C. The rapid assessment for a medical patient is directed toward the patient's chief complaint. The clothing may be removed in the area assessed, but all of the patient's clothes do not need to be removed. A head-to-toe assessment may be indicated if the patient is unresponsive. The rapid assessment will help identify trauma but cannot rule it out. p. 180, Objectives 3, 4

21. D. The rapid trauma assessment should be performed on unresponsive medical patients to try to find signs of trauma or medical conditions. The trauma assessment should be performed if there is suspected trauma. The patient should be immobilized unless you can be sure the patient has no spinal injury. p. 182, Objective 4

22. B. The detailed physical examination is designed for trauma patients who have been seriously injured and who may have hidden injuries. The examination is slower and more methodical than the focused history and physical examination. The detailed physical examination ideally should be performed en route to the receiving facility. The detailed physical examination can be performed on medical patients but is primarily for trauma patients. p. 188, Objective 4

23. C. Medical patients who are unresponsive should receive a detailed physical examination to try to find clues about their condition. Responsive medical patients without injuries do not routinely receive a detailed physical examination. Patients with an isolated injury do not require a detailed physical examination. p. 188, Objective 4

24. A. While performing the detailed physical examination of the head, evaluate the ears and nose for drainage, the eyes for discoloration, and the mouth for foreign bodies. The pupils and stability of the face are assessed the first time during the focused history and physical examination, and the mouth is examined for any airway obstructions during the initial assessment. These steps are repeated in the detailed physical examination. p. 89, Objectives 1, 2

25. D. The neck should be assessed for trauma and jugular vein distention. Breath sounds are assessed in four places: bilaterally at the apices and the bases of the lungs. The abdomen is assessed in all four quadrants. The pelvis should not be evaluated if there is any sign of injury or if the patient complains of pain in the pelvis. p. 190, Objective 2

26. B. When assessing the extremities, assess for distal pulse, motor function, and sensation, besides DCAP-BTLS. p. 192, Objective 2

27. D. The ongoing assessment allows the EMT–Basic to document trends in the patient's condition. Vital signs are evaluated every time the ongoing assessment is repeated. The initial assessment is repeated during the ongoing assessment. The ongoing assessment is repeated based on the patient's condition. p. 199, Objective 2

28. C. The ongoing assessment is repeated every 15 minutes for stable patients and every 5 minutes for unstable patients. p. 200, Objective 2

29. B. The ongoing assessment should be repeated one last time about 5 minutes away from the receiving facility, so you can report a recent assessment at bedside. If an intervention is inadequate, it should be corrected immediately. Pupil size and mental status are assessment findings, not interventions. Whether the patient is responsive or unresponsive, the entire ongoing assessment should be repeated, including the focused history and physical examination. p. 201, Objective 2

30. C. The FCC, or Federal Communications Commission, regulates radio frequencies and is responsible for assigning radio channels, licensing radio operators, and routinely monitoring radio transmissions. p. 208, Objective 1

31. A. The medical direction physician with whom you talk may be at the receiving facility or at another location. Orders from medical direction should be repeated back to the physician word for word to check accuracy. If the order is unclear, ask questions until you are sure of the order. Reports to medical direction should be concise and organized so they may understand the patient's condition quickly. p. 209, Objective 3

32. C. Everyday language is less confusing than codes and should be used for radio communications. The microphone should be 5 to 7 cm from your mouth when transmitting. Speak clearly and slowly to minimize confusion. Words that are difficult to hear such as "yes" and "no," should be avoided. p. 208, Objective 2

33. B. A repeater is a remote receiver that receives a transmission from a lower portable and transmits the signal at a higher power. A base station is a stationary radio with superior transmitting and receiving capabilities. Encoders and decoders can be used to block out radio transmissions not intended for a particular unit. p. 207

34. C. EMT–Basics should notify dispatch when: receiving the call, responding to the call, arriving at the scene, arriving at the patient's side, leaving the scene for the receiving facility, arriving at the receiving facility, leaving the hospital for the station, and arriving at the station. Information regarding the patient's status is not routinely communicated with dispatch. Notify dispatch when arriving at the receiving facility, not after giving bedside report. p. 210, Objective 9

35. B. Administrative information includes the incident location, the type of location, the date the incident was reported, the time the incident was reported, the date the EMS unit was notified, the time the EMS unit was notified, the time the unit responded, the time of arrival at the scene, the time of arrival at the patient, time the EMS unit left the scene, time of the EMS arrival at the destination, time of transfer of patient care, time the EMS unit was back in service, the use of lights and siren to and from the scene, and the crew members responding to the scene. p. 219, Objective 1

36. A. The type of location is part of the administrative information. The patient information includes: age and gender; chief complaint; cause of injury; preexisting conditions; signs and symptoms present; injury description; level of responsiveness; pulse rate; respiratory rate; systolic blood pressure in patients 3 years of age or older; skin perfusion; skin color, temperature, and condition; procedures performed on the patient; medications administered; and response to treatment. p. 219, Objective 1

37. C. The prehospital care report can be used for case reviews or continuing education if the patient's confidentiality is protected. Care reports can be released for billing purposes to other healthcare professionals assuming care for the patient. The prehospital care report should contain only objective information. EMT–Basics should treat the patient based on signs and symptoms present and not make a diagnosis. p. 220

38. C. The correct abbreviation for nothing by mouth is NPO. For a list of common medical abbreviations, refer to page 224 in Mosby's EMT–Basic textbook. p. 224

39. D. Situations such as infectious disease exposure, injury to EMT–Basics or bystanders, equipment damage or malfunction, vehicle crashes involving the response unit, patient refusals, abuse or neglect,

crime scenes, or hazardous materials incidents should be documented on a special report form. Documentation errors should have a single line drawn through them, with the correct information printed beside the incorrect information. Initial beside the correction. Refusals should be carefully documented, with a witness other than your partner signing the refusal form. Be careful to document only the care that was given, even if you know you left out important care. p. 228, Objective 4

● CHAPTER 16
GENERAL PHARMACOLOGY

● MATCHING

1. H
2. D
3. F
4. K
5. B
6. A
7. G
8. C
9. J
10. E
11. I

Definitions to key terms can be found on page 235 of the student textbook.

● REVIEW QUESTIONS

1. False. Pharmacology is the science of drugs and includes the study of their origin, ingredients, uses, and actions on the body. A medication is any substance that alters the body's functions when taken into the body. Medication and drug are two words often used interchangeably. p. 236

2. EMT–Basics carry the medications *oxygen*, *activated charcoal*, and *oral glucose* on the EMS unit. EMT–Basics may assist patients with their physician-prescribed nitroglycerin, prescribed inhaler, or epinephrine autoinjector. p. 237, Objectives 1, 3

3. A. The manufacturer assigns the medication its trade name. The generic name is usually a simple form of the chemical name, listed in the *U.S. Pharmacopeia*. p. 237, Objectives 2, 4

4. True. Because more than one company may manufacture a drug, it may have more than one trade name. p. 237, Objectives 2, 4

5. EMT–Basics will commonly deal with medications in the form of a suspension, gel, gas, fine powder for inhalation, compressed powders or tablets, sublingual spray, and liquid for injection. The route of administration will affect the speed of absorption of the drug. p. 238, Objective 5

6. Match the generic name in Column 1 with the trade name in Column 2: 1. *c;* 2. *b;* 3. *d;* 4. *a.* p. 238, Objectives 2, 4

7. True. A contraindication is any factor that makes a medication unsafe to administer or a procedure unsafe to perform. Contraindications apply to a situation when a medication should not be used, because it will be of little benefit or potential harm. p. 239

8. A. The dose of a medication may depend on the patient's age or weight, or there may be one standard dose for all patients. Factors such as gender, race and height do not affect the medication dose. p. 239

9. False. Oral medications cannot be delivered to unresponsive patients, because the patient must be alert enough to swallow. Oral medications administered to an unresponsive patient may cause an airway obstruction. p. 240

10. B. When medications are administered sublingually, the medication is absorbed by the capillaries under the tongue, bypassing the digestive tract. p. 240

11. D. Epinephrine autoinjectors deliver medication through the intramuscular route. The medication is absorbed into the tissues and then into the bloodstream. p. 240

12. The undesirable actions of a medication are called *side effects.* The known side effects of a medication should be anticipated when the EMT–Basic administers the drug. p. 241

13. True. Many medications have predictable side effects. By knowing the pharmacology of a medication, EMT–Basics may be able to anticipate side effects and be prepared for them. p. 241

14. After administering a medication, carefully monitor the patient for *desired effects* and *side effects.* Report any findings to the receiving facility and document them in your prehospital care report. p. 241

15. **a.** EMT–Basics typically carry the medications: oral glucose, activated charcoal, and oxygen. p. 236. **b.** EMT–Basics can assist a patient with his/her prescribed inhaler; nitroglycerin; epinephrine autoinjector. p. 237. **c.** An indication is the most common use of a medication for treating a specific illness or condition—signs and symptoms for when a medication is used. A contraindication is a situation in which a medication should not be used. A dose is the amount of the medication that should be administered. p. 239

● **CHAPTER 17**
RESPIRATORY EMERGENCIES

● **REVIEW QUESTIONS**

1. **a.** Pharynx; **b.** Nasopharynx; **c.** Oropharynx; **d.** Epiglottis; **e.** Larynx; **f.** Trachea; **g.** Right bronchus; **h.** Diaphragm; **i.** Left bronchus. p. 247, Objective 1

2. True. Carbon dioxide is given up from the body and oxygen is absorbed into the body through the alveoli. p. 247, Objective 1

3. A. Inhaled air contains high concentrations of oxygen, whereas exhaled air contains high concentrations of carbon dioxide. p. 247, Objective 1

4. C. The normal respiratory rate for a child is 15 to 30 breaths per minute. The normal rate for an adult is 12 to 20 breaths per minute and for an infant 25 to 50 breaths per minute. These are average respiratory rates. A patient may be breathing slower or faster and still be within his/her normal limits. p. 248, Objective 7

5. Adequate breathing means the patient has a normal rate, rhythm, *chest expansion*, and *tidal volume*. p. 248, Objective 7

6. True. A rate that is too fast or too slow may cause the patient to receive less oxygen than the body needs. p. 249, Objective 2

7. Any change in the patient's breathing may cause there to be inadequate oxygen available to the cells. p. 249, Objective 1

8. D. The ability to speak in full sentences does not indicate respiratory distress. Patients in respiratory distress often have difficulty saying more than a few words before taking a breath. p. 250, Objective 2

9. False. Normal breathing should be silent. Noises made during breathing can be signs of respiratory difficulty. p. 250, Objective 2

10. General signs and symptoms of difficulty breathing include: shortness of breath; restlessness or anxiety; patient position; altered mental status; abdominal breathing; increased or decreased breathing rate; and increased pulse rate. Visual signs and symptoms of difficulty breathing include: changes in skin color, temperature, or condition; unusual anatomy; or retractions/use of accessory muscles. Auditory signs and symptoms of breathing difficulty include: noisy breathing; inability to speak due to breathing efforts; coughing; irregular breathing rhythm; or unequal breath sounds. p. 250, Objective 2

11. True. Changes in a patient's anatomy can occur over long periods of respiratory problems, such as a barrel chest. p. 250, Objective 2

12. The acronym OPQRST is used during the focused history and physical examination and stands for Onset, Provocation, Quality, Radiation, Signs and Symptoms, and Time. p. 251, Objective 3

13. False. Responsive patients with no suspected trauma should be transported in the position of comfort. Patients with difficulty breathing often cannot tolerate lying flat and prefer to sit upright. p. 250, Objectives 3, 5

14. The first medication to administer to a patient in respiratory distress is *oxygen.* p. 252, Objectives 3, 5

15. False. EMTs can assist patients with their prescribed inhaler only if the patients have their own medication prescribed to them by a physician. p. 253, Objectives 6, 8

16. B. Inhalers are used to dilate bronchioles and decrease resistance inside the airways. Decreased resistance makes it easier for the patient to breathe. p. 253, Objective 8

17. Albuterol and isoetharine are *generic* names for the medication in an inhaler. p. 253, Objective 8

18. To use an inhaler, patients must: 1) have signs and symptoms of difficulty breathing; 2) have their own physician-prescribed inhaler; and 3) the EMT must obtain permission from medical direction to help with the administration of the medication. p. 254, Objectives 4, 5, 8

19. Contraindications for the use of a prescribed inhaler include: a patient who is not oriented enough to use the device properly; a patient using an inhaler that was prescribed for someone else; the patient has already taken the maximum recommended dose; medical direction has not granted permission. p. 254, Objective 8

20. False. A spacer is a device used to help a patient to get the maximum effect from the medication. If the patient has a spacer, it should be used. p. 254, Objective 8

21. False. Infants and very young children generally lack the coordination to use an inhaler. p. 254, Objectives 6, 9

22. A. Possible side effects of prescribed inhalers include increased pulse rate, tremors, nervousness, and sometimes nausea. p. 254, Objective 8

23. Number the following steps for assisting with a prescribed inhaler in the proper order: 6—Hold breath as long as comfortable; 1—Check expiration date; 3—Remove oxygen mask, patient exhales deeply; 2—Shake vigorously; 5—Begin inhalation, depress inhaler; 4—Place mouth over inhaler mouthpiece. p. 255, Objective 6

24. **a.** General signs and symptoms of difficulty breathing include shortness of breath, restlessness or anxiety, patient position, altered mental status, use of accessory muscles, abdominal breathing, increased or decreased breathing. Case 17A Answers: rate, and increased pulse rate. p. 250. **b.** Using OPQRST, you would attempt to ascertain if there is a history of respiratory problems; what makes it better or worse; is there associated pain; severity of distress; when it started and how long it lasted; and if the patient takes any medication for breathing problems. Also, SAMPLE history should be included: signs and symptoms, allergies, medications, past pertinent history, last oral intake, and events leading to the event. p. 251. **c.** Allow the patient to assume a position of comfort. Most patients will prefer to sit upright to make breathing easier. p. 253

25. **a.** Common trade names include Proventil, Ventolin, Bronkosol, Bronkometer, Alupent, and Metaprel. **b.** The medication is absorbed into the tissues of the lungs, generally dilating the bronchioles to decrease resistance inside the airways. p. 253. **c.** You should obtain a brief pertinent history of past and present illness and how many doses of the inhaler the child took before you arrived. p. 253. **d.** 1) The patient must have signs and symptoms of a respiratory emergency. 2) The patient must have his/her own physician-prescribed inhaler. 3) You must obtain specific authorization from medical direction to aid the patient in inhaled medication administration through either on- or off-line medical direction. p. 254

● CHAPTER 18
CARDIOVASCULAR EMERGENCIES

● MATCHING

1. I
2. F
3. A
4. B
5. G
6. H
7. D
8. C
9. E

Definitions to key terms can be found on page 259 of the student textbook.

10. p. 261

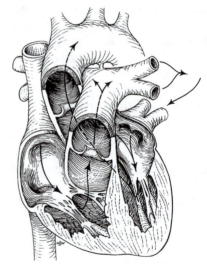

From McKenna/Sanders: *Workbook to Accompany Mosby's Paramedic Textbook,* 1994, Mosby Lifeline.

● REVIEW QUESTIONS

1. True. The two upper chambers of the heart are called the atria, the two lower chambers are called

the ventricles, and there are valves between the chambers to prevent the backflow of blood. p. 260, Objective 1

2. Match the arteries in Column 1 with the correct location in Column 2: 1. *e*; 2. *c*; 3. *d*; 4. *h*; 5. *f*; 6. *b*; 7. *g*; 8. *a*. p. 262, Objective 1

3. A. Blood from the vena cava enters the right atrium, then the right ventricle, to be pumped to the lungs to be reoxygenated. p. 262, Objective 1

4. Blood contains plasma, red cells, white cells, and *platelets*. p. 262, Objective 1

5. True. The contraction of the ventricles causes a wave of blood to be sent through the body, generating a pulse. p. 262, Objective 1

6. Central pulses can be palpated at the carotid and femoral arteries. Peripheral pulses can be located at the radial, brachial, dorsalis pedis, and posterior tibial arteries. p. 263, Objective 1

7. C. The first number in a blood pressure is the systolic value, measuring the pressure in the arteries when the heart contracts, and the second number is the diastolic value, measuring the pressure in the arteries when the heart relaxes. p. 263, Objective 1

8. Another term used to describe shock is *hypoperfusion*. p. 263, Objective 1

9. B. High blood pressure is not an indicator of shock. Signs and symptoms of shock (hypoperfusion) include rapid and weak pulse; pale or cyanotic skin; cool, clammy skin; rapid and shallow breathing; restlessness and anxiety; mental dullness, confusion; nausea, vomiting and thirst; low or decreasing blood pressure (usually a late sign); and subnormal temperature. p. 263, Objective 1

10. Chest pressure or discomfort that usually goes away with rest is called *angina*. p. 264, Objective 2

11. B. When muscles can no longer get oxygen, they become ischemic, which causes pain. p. 264, Objective 2

12. Respiratory pain is often *sharp or stabbing* and *increases* with breathing. Cardiac pain is usually *crushing, dull, or pressure* and *does not change* with movement. p. 264, Objective 2

13. Cardiac pain can radiate anywhere in the body but commonly radiates to the shoulder, neck, or jaw. p. 264, Objective 2

14. Severity can be measured on a scale of 1 to 10 with 10 being the *worst* pain. p. 265, Objective 2

15. The acronym OPQRST can be used to evaluate a patient's signs and symptoms. O stands for onset, P for provocation, Q for quality, R for radiation, S for severity, T for time. p. 265, Objective 2

16. The first medication delivered to the cardiac patient is *oxygen*. p. 265, Objective 2

17. Responsive medical patients should be transported in the position of comfort. Most patients prefer to sit up when they are experiencing chest pain or difficulty breathing. p. 265, Objective 7

18. False. Nitroglycerin only can be administered after an initial assessment and focused history and physical examination, and with permission from medical direction. p. 265, Objectives 40, 41

19. B. Nitroglycerin dilates blood vessels, allowing more blood to flow through them. Administration of nitroglycerin may cause a drop in blood pressure. p. 265, Objective 41

20. Nitroglycerin is contraindicated when 1) the patient's blood pressure is less than 100 mm Hg, 2) the patient does not have his/her own physician-prescribed nitroglycerin, 3) the patient has a head injury or is not alert, 4) the patient is an infant or child, or 5) the patient has received the maximum dose. p. 266, Objective 42

21. A. Nitroglycerin does not commonly cause muscle tremors. Common side effects include lower blood pressure, headache, pulse rate changes, and burning sensation under the tongue. p. 266, Objective 42

22. The primary intervention that makes the most difference in survival from cardiac arrest is *early defibrillation*. p. 268, Objectives 10, 11

23. C. Ventricular fibrillation is the condition in which the heart is not contracting effectively and is quivering. p. 269

24. C. The AED should only be placed on patients who are in cardiac arrest. The EMT should confirm that the patient is pulseless, apneic, and unresponsive. p. 269, Objectives 3, 12, 18

25. True. The EMT performing the defibrillation must make sure that no one is in contact with the patient or the stretcher before delivering the shock. p. 270, Objective 4

26. C. CPR can be stopped for up to 90 seconds while the patient is being defibrillated. p. 270, Objective 20

27. A patient must weigh at least *90* pounds and be at least *12* years of age before the AED can be used. p. 270, Objectives 3, 6

28. A. A maximum of six shocks can be delivered before beginning to prepare the patient for transport. Medical direction may advise more or less shocks before transport. p. 274, Objectives 26, 27

29. False. Do not assess the patient between the first three shocks. Check the pulse after each set of stacked shocks and periodically while performing CPR. p. 275 , Objective 29

30. **a.** Angina is the discomfort felt when the heart does not receive enough oxygen. It is commonly experienced after exertion, and the patient usually feels better with rest. p. 264. **b.** The indications for nitroglycerin include signs and symptoms of cardiac chest pain; patient has physician-prescribed sublingual tablets or spray; EMT–Basic has approval from medical direction. p. 264. **c.** Contradictions for nitroglycerin administration include: patient has a systolic blood pressure less than 100 mm Hg; patient does not have own

nitroglycerin that is prescribed by a medical doctor; patient has a head injury or is not mentally alert; patient is an infant or child; patient has already taken the maximum prescribed dosage prior to EMS arrival. p. 266

31. **a.** Common signs and symptoms for cardiac compromise include: squeezing, dull pressure or pain in the chest that radiates to the arms, neck, jaw, or upper back; sudden onset of sweating; difficulty breathing; anxiety or irritability; feeling of impending doom; abnormal and sometimes irregular pulse rate; abnormal blood pressure; epigastric pain; nausea or vomiting. p. 264. **b.** No. The medication was not prescribed for this patient. p. 266

32. **a.** AEDs will recognize ventricular fibrillation and ventricular tachycardia as shockable rhythms. p. 269. **b.** One electrode is placed to the right of the upper portion of the sternum below the clavicle. The other electrode is placed over the ribs to the left of the nipple with the center in the midaxillary line. p. 271. **c.** The AED will deliver up to three stacked shocks per cycle. **d.** The progressive energy levels are 200, 200 to 300, and 360 joules. p. 275

● CHAPTER 19
DIABETES AND ALTERED MENTAL STATUS

● MATCHING

1. F
2. D
3. E
4. A
5. B
6. C

Definitions to key terms can be found on page 283 of the student textbook.

● REVIEW QUESTIONS

1. False. Altered mental status can be caused by medical conditions such as hypoglycemia or seizures or by trauma such as trauma to the head. p. 284

2. Signs and symptoms of hypoglycemia include slurred speech; unresponsiveness; appearance of intoxication or taking drugs; increased heart rate; cool, clammy skin; and combativeness. p. 285, Objective 1

3. True. Not all seizures cause the body to convulse. p. 285

4. Common causes of seizures include: fever, infection, poisoning, intoxication, hypoglycemia, head trauma, decreased levels of oxygen, epilepsy uncontrolled by medication, or no known cause. p. 285

5. False. Not all seizures are life threatening. p. 285

6. One of the most common causes of seizures in children is a *fever*. p. 285

7. The time following a seizure when the patient may be disoriented is called the *postictal* period. p. 286

8. Common causes of altered mental status include: low blood sugar, seizure, poisoning, intoxication, infection, head trauma, decreased oxygen levels, and hypothermia or hyperthermia. p. 286, Objective 1

9. The primary goal of emergency treatment for patients with altered mental status is maintaining an *open airway*. p. 287, Objective 3

10. Major points to assess during the focused history and physical examination of a patient with altered mental status include the onset, duration, associated signs and symptoms, evidence of trauma, seizures, and fever. p. 287, Objectives 1, 2

11. True. Evaluating the scene can reveal signs of trauma or evidence of a medical condition (such as a medic alert bracelet or medications). p. 287

12. C. Patients with altered mental status are considered unstable and their vital signs should be evaluated every 5 minutes. p. 287, Objective 2

13. Ask patients with a history of diabetes when their last meal was and whether they have taken their medications. p. 287, Objective 2

14. False. Oral glucose is only indicated for patients with an altered mental status and a history of diabetes. The patient must be alert enough to swallow so the glucose does not cause an airway obstruction. p. 289, Objective 4

15. True. The patient must be alert enough to swallow so the oral glucose does not cause airway compromise. p. 189, Objectives 2, 3

16. A. Oral glucose is a generic name. Trade names include Insta-Glucose and Glutose. p. 189, Objective 4

17. False. The medication should be administered by a tongue depressor placed between the patient's cheek and gums to be absorbed. p. 289, Objective 4

18. Absence of a *gag reflex* is a contraindication for administration of oral glucose. p. 289, Objective 4

19. Oral glucose improves the patient's condition by increasing *blood sugar*. p. 289, Objective 4

20. True. Medical direction must be involved with the administration of any medication to a patient, including oral glucose. p. 289, Objective 5

21. **a.** Hypoglycemia. If your partner takes her insulin but does not eat, the insulin will draw on other stores of sugar in the body tissues. p. 285. **b.** Altered mental status, cold and clammy skin, hostility or agitation, anxiety, combative behavior (in extreme cases), and seizures are all signs and symptoms of a diabetic emergency. p. 285. **c.** Request the dispatcher to respond another EMS unit to the crash scene. Contact medical direction to obtain an order for oral glucose. As long as she

remains responsive, you may administer the full tube of glucose between your partner's cheek and gum, allowing the mucous membrane to absorb the glucose. p. 289

22. **a.** You should perform an initial assessment that includes assessing the level of responsiveness, position the patient (with spinal precautions), and check airway, breathing, and circulation. p. 287. **b.** Common causes of altered mental status include: low blood sugar; seizure; poisoning; intoxication; infection; head trauma; decreased oxygen levels; hypothermia or hyperthermia. p. 286. **c.** Assess the scene for additional clues; obtain baseline vital signs and monitor them every 5 minutes; check the patient for medical identification tags; maintain airway and ventilation; rapidly transport for physician evaluation. p. 287

● **CHAPTER 20**
ALLERGIC REACTIONS

● **REVIEW QUESTIONS**

1. D. Allergic reactions are exaggerated immune responses to an allergen. Reactions can be severe, causing hypoperfusion and respiratory difficulty, or minor, involving only a local reaction. p. 294, Objective 1

2. False. Some allergic reactions are mild, others can be life threatening. The type of reaction depends on the allergen involved and the individual patient. p. 194, Objectives 2, 7

3. Common allergens include food (shellfish, crustaceans, peanuts), plants (poison ivy), medications (penicillin, aspirin), and environmental factors (dust, pollen). p. 294, Objective 1

4. Common signs and symptoms of an allergic reaction include: itchy, watery eyes; coughing or stridor; wheezing; rapid, labored breathing; headache; runny nose; tightness in the throat; increased heart rate; decreased blood pressure; itchy, red, or flushed skin; hives; and swelling. p. 295, Objective 4

5. Itchy, watery eyes; runny nose; and a headache are all signs and symptoms of a *mild* allergic reaction. p. 295, Objective 7

6. The first sign of hypoperfusion may be a change in *mental status*. p. 296, Objective 1

7. Altered mental status is caused by decreased *blood flow* to the tissues. This results in too little oxygen being delivered to the tissues. p. 296, Objective 4

8. B. Signs and symptoms of hypoperfusion (including low blood pressure) and respiratory compromise are signs of a true medical emergency. p. 296, Objective 7

9. B. The epinephrine autoinjector is used for patients with severe allergic reactions. p. 297, Objective 5

10. A patient with an allergic reaction and signs of respiratory compromise should be assessed every 5 minutes. p. 297, Objective 2

11. A. Epinephrine works by dilating the bronchioles, making breathing easier, and constricting the blood vessels, increasing blood pressure. p. 297, Objective 5

12. To use an autoinjector, the patient must have a severe allergic reaction (with respiratory distress and/or hypoperfusion), have medication prescribed by the patient's own physician, and medical direction must authorize the use. p. 297, Objective 5

13. False. When the patient is experiencing a life-threatening reaction, there are no contraindications to the use of the autoinjector. All of the indications listed in question 12 must be met. p. 297, Objective 5

14. True. An autoinjector is designed to be used by people who are not familiar with calculating drug dosages and giving injections. The medication is automatically injected at the right dose when the needle is depressed against the thigh. p. 298, Objective 5

15. C. Epinephrine does not typically cause sleepiness. Common side effects of epinephrine include increased heart rate, pale skin, dizziness, chest pain, headache, nausea and vomiting, excitability, and anxiousness. p. 298, Objective 5

16. False. Airway management is always a priority in patient care. p. 299, Objective 3

17. **a.** Signs and symptoms of allergic reactions include: itchy, watery eyes; coughing or stridor; wheezing; rapid labored respirations; headache; runny nose; tightness in the throat; increased heart rate; decreased blood pressure; itchy, red, or flushed skin; hives; and swelling. p. 296. **b.** To use the epinephrine autoinjector, you will need assessment findings of a severe allergic reaction, the patient must have his/her own physician-prescribed medication, and you will need authorization from medical direction. p. 297. **c.** To administer the autoinjector: remove the safety cap on the autoinjector; place the tip of the autoinjector at a 90° angle against the lateral portion of the patient's thigh midway between the waist and the knee; push the injector firmly against the thigh and hold the injector in place for at least 10 seconds or until the medication is injected; dispose of the injector in a bio-hazard container. p. 298

18. **a.** Insect bites, foods, plants, medications, chemicals, dust, and pollen all can cause mild allergic reactions. p. 294. **b.** Any assessment findings that reveal hypoperfusion (such as cool, clammy skin, an elevated heart rate, or decreased blood pressure) or respiratory distress (such as coughing or stridor, tightness in the throat, or rapid labored

breathing) would indicate a severe allergic reaction. p. 296. **c.** No. She has no physician-prescribed autoinjector. The patient is not wheezing and has no signs of respiratory compromise or hypoperfusion. p. 297

● CHAPTER 21
POISONING AND OVERDOSE

● MATCHING
1. C
2. F
3. D
4. E
5. B
6. A

Definitions to key terms can be found on page 303 of the student textbook.

● REVIEW QUESTIONS
1. True. Any medication can cause a poisoning if a larger dose than recommended is taken. p. 304, Objective 1
2. Ongoing assessments are every *5* minutes for unstable patients and every *15* minutes for stable patients. p. 304, Objectives 3, 4
3. When assessing the poisoning or overdose patient, ask the following questions in addition to the questions you would normally ask during the focused history and physical examination for medical patients: What substance was involved?; When did you ingest or become exposed to the substance?; If you ingested the poison, how much did you ingest?; Over what time period did the poisoning occur?; What has happened since the poisoning?; and How much do you weigh? p. 305, Objectives 3, 4
4. True. An overdose can be an intentional use of too much medication, or it could be accidental. Patients who are taking many medications can be confused as to the dose for each, and may make mistakes in the doses. p. 305, Objective 1
5. B. Knowing the amount of time over which the patient was exposed to a toxin will help medical direction determine treatment options for prehospital personnel and in-hospital care. p. 305, Objectives 3, 4
6. False. Over-the-counter treatments may not be appropriate depending on the type of poison involved. When contacting medical direction, advise them if the patient has taken any home remedies. p. 305, Objectives 3, 4
7. B. Ingested toxins commonly cause nausea, vomiting, and diarrhea but can also cause altered men-

tal status, abdominal pain, chemical burns around the mouth, and particular breath odors. p. 305, Objectives 1, 2
8. Any pills or tablets in the mouth should be removed so that no further medication is absorbed and to prevent airway compromise. The EMT–Basic should use gloved hands to remove the pills from the mouth of an unresponsive patient and insert a bite block in the patient's mouth so the EMT–Basic is not bitten. p. 305, Objectives 3, 5
9. Inhaled toxins can cause difficulty breathing, chest pain, coughing, hoarseness, dizziness, headache, confusion, seizures, and altered mental status. p. 306, Objectives 1, 4
10. The primary treatment for inhaled poisoning is *oxygen*. After assuring the scene is safe for you and the patient, begin to administer oxygen at 15 L/min via a nonrebreather mask. p. 306, Objective 4
11. D. Injected toxins cause weakness, dizziness, chills, fever, nausea, and vomiting, as well as local irritation at the injection site. p. 307, Objectives 1, 3, 4
12. D. Injected poisons can reach the body by bites or stings or by intravenous, intramuscular, or subcutaneous injection. The sublingual route means that the substance was absorbed by the capillaries under the tongue. p. 307, Objective 1
13. False. In the case of injection poisonings, the animal that caused the bite or sting can also be dangerous to the rescuer, and you should not attempt to capture the animal. p. 307, Objective 4
14. B. The gender of the patient will not affect absorption rates. The blood flow to the area will greatly influence the absorption rate. p. 307, Objective 1
15. C. Absorbed toxins are substances that come in contact with the skin and are absorbed into the body. p. 307, Objective 1
16. A. Dry substances should be brushed away from the skin, liquid substances irrigated for at least 20 minutes. Contact medical direction or consult the container for directions for dealing with accidental skin contact. p. 307, Objective 4
17. B. Activated charcoal is an oral medication and is only effective for ingested toxins. p. 311, Objective 6
18. Activated charcoal works by *binding* to the toxin in the *stomach*. The medication is therefore not absorbed into the bloodstream through the digestive system. p. 311, Objective 6
19. A. Activated charcoal is the generic name, and LiquiChar and InstaChar are examples of trade names for the drug. p. 311, Objective 6
20. Contraindications to the use of activated charcoal include: 1) a patient with an altered mental status, 2) suspected ingestion of an acid or alkali substance, 3) inability to swallow, or 4) seizures. p. 311, Objective 6
21. False. Activated charcoal is designed to bind to toxins in the stomach. If the patient vomits, med-

ical direction may order another dose of activated charcoal. p. 311, Objective 7

22. **a.** The normal dose of activated charcoal for infants and children is 1 g per kilogram of body weight or 12.5 to 25 g. p. 311. **b.** The indication for activated charcoal is a patient with clinical signs and symptoms of ingested poisonings. Contra-indications are an altered mental status, suspected ingestion of an acid or alkali substance, inability to swallow, seizures. p. 311. **c.** Contact medical direction. The physician may order that the dose be repeated one time.

23. **a.** After controlling the airway, oxygen is the first treatment. p. 306. **b.** Carbon monoxide is an invisible, odorless, and tasteless gas. General symptoms of exposure may include weakness, sleepiness, headache, dizziness, or confusion. p. 306. **c.** Carbon monoxide poisoning is a serious possibility with fire victims. p. 306

● CHAPTER 22
ENVIRONMENTAL EMERGENCIES

● MATCHING

1. D
2. E
3. F
4. B
5. G
6. C
7. A

Definitions to key terms can be found on page 315 of the student textbook.

● REVIEW QUESTIONS

1. True. Any significant changes in body temperature can affect the functioning of the body. p. 316, Objective 2

2. The human body loses heat by evaporation, conduction, radiation, *convection*, and *respiration*. p. 316, Objective 1

3. When body temperature begins to decrease, the body produces heat by *shivering*. p. 317, Objective 2

4. When body temperature begins to increase, the body produces *sweat*, which cools the body by evaporation. p. 317, Objective 4

5. True. Any drop below the normal temperature is classified as hypothermia. p. 317, Objective 1

6. False. The most common cause of generalized hypothermia is exposure to cold environment. p. 317, Objective 1

7. Predisposing factors for generalized hypothermia include: cold environments; immersion in water; age; alcohol; shock; head or spinal cord injury;

burns; generalized infection; diabetes; hypoglycemia; and some medications and poisons. p. 317

8. An unreliable sign of hypothermia is cool *extremities*. Blood flow to the extremities is usually limited when the body is trying to preserve heat. p. 318, Objective 2

9. Cool *abdominal skin* is a sign of a generalized cold emergency. p. 318, Objective 2

10. C. Slow respirations occur later in hypothermia. Signs and symptoms of early hypothermia include rapid pulse, normal blood pressure, rapid breathing, red skin, reactive pupils, and shivering. p. 318, Objective 2

11. True. By increasing the body's functions, the body attempts to produce heat. p. 319, Objective 2

12. Allowing the body to produce its own heat while preventing further heat loss is passive rewarming. Adding heat to the body is active rewarming. p. 319, Objective 3

13. Heat packs at the axilla and groin are a form of *active* rewarming. p. 319, Objective 3

14. False. Rewarming a patient in late hypothermia can cause lethal arrhythmias. Simply prevent heat loss in the patient and transport gently to the receiving facility. p. 320, Objective 3

15. A pulse check for a severely hypothermic patient should be between *30* and *45* seconds. p. 321, Objective 3

16. Five body areas most susceptible to localized cold injuries are the fingers, toes, ears, nose, and face. p. 321, Objective 2

17. C. A tingling sensation occurs in early local cold injuries. Late local cold injuries usually involve a loss of sensation. p. 321, Objective 2

18. False. Rubbing and massaging a cold area can cause serious tissue damage. p. 322, Objective 3

19. Predisposing factors for heat emergencies include: hot, humid weather; vigorous activity; elderly patients; infants and newborns; heart disease; dehydration; obesity; previous history of hyperthermia; fever; fatigue; diabetes; and drugs and medications. p. 322, Objective 4

20. True. A sign of a severe heat emergency exists anytime the patient has hot skin, either dry or moist. p. 323, Objective 4

21. D. When the patient has hot skin, all measures to cool the body should be used, including fanning the patient and turning up the air conditioning, keeping the skin wet, and applying cold packs. p. 324, Objective 5

22. Drowning is defined as death following immersion in water. Near drowning means the patient survived an immersion incident. p. 324, Objective 6

23. Patients found unresponsive in the water should be treated and evaluated for possible *spinal* injury. p. 324, Objective 7

24. Bites and stings may cause localized reactions but may also produce an *allergic* reaction. p. 325, Objective 8

25. False. As with any patient, the first priority in the management of a patient with a bite or sting is to assess and manage airway, breathing, and circulation. p. 325, Objective 8

26. B. Extremities with bite or sting injuries should be positioned slightly below the level of the heart. p. 325, Objective 8

27. True. Use a credit card or similar material to scape the stinger out of the skin. Do not squeeze a stinger with tweezers because this may cause additional venom to be injected into the patient. p. 325, Objective 8

28. **a.** Predisposing factors for generalized hypothermia include: cold environments; immersion in water; extremes of age; alcohol consumption; shock; head or spinal cord injury; burns; generalized infection; diabetes; hypoglycemia; and some medications and poisons. p. 318. **b.** Hypothermic patients often exhibit poor coordination; memory disturbances; reduced or absent sensation of touch; mood changes; joint or muscle pain; poor judgement; less communicative; dizziness; and speech difficulties. p. 318. **c.** You should remove the patient from the cold environment and protect the patient from further heat loss. Remove any wet clothing and cover the patient with a blanket. You should avoid rough handling, administer high-flow oxygen, not allow the patient to eat or drink stimulants, not massage the extremities; and check for a pulse for 30 to 45 seconds before starting CPR. p. 320

29. **a.** Immobilize the spine if trauma is suspected; ensure an adequate airway; artificially ventilate the patient with supplemental oxygen; and suction as needed. p. 324. **b.** Place the patient on the left side (or tilt the long backboard to the left). With suction immediately available, place your hand over the epigastric area and apply firm pressure to relieve the distention. p. 324. **c.** No. Do not attempt to relieve gastric distention unless it interferes with artificial ventilation. There is a significant risk of aspiration. p. 324

● **CHAPTER 23**
BEHAVIORAL EMERGENCIES

● **MATCHING**

1. D
2. E
3. A
4. B
5. C

Definitions to key terms can be found on page 329 of the student textbook. Key terms cover Objective 1.

● **REVIEW QUESTIONS**

1. The way in which people act on a day-to-day basis is called their *behavior*. p. 330, Objective 1

2. A person's behavior can be altered by many factors, including: situational stress; alcohol, legal and illegal drugs; illness; diabetes; hypoxia; hypoperfusion; thermoregulatory emergencies; and trauma. p. 330, Objectives 2, 3

3. B. Treat patients who are not thinking rationally carefully and calmly. Do not excite or agitate these patients. p. 331, Objective 8

4. Risk factors for suicide include patients who: are more than 40 years of age; are widowed or divorced; are alcoholic; are depressed; have a previous history of self-destructive behavior; have a serious illness; have an unusual gathering of destructive articles; have suffered the recent loss of a loved one; have recent arrests or imprisonment; and have recently lost a job. p. 331, Objective 4

5. False. Patients who commit suicide may display no risk factors, and people with many risk factors for suicide may never consider killing themselves. p. 332, Objective 4

6. True. Scene size-up, including scene safety, is the most important aspect of entering any potentially violent or dangerous scene. p. 332, Objective 6

7. A. Signs of potential violence include sitting on the edge of the chair; clenched fists; yelling and using profanity; throwing things; standing or moving toward the EMT–Basic; holding onto a potentially dangerous object; and behavior that makes the EMT–Basic uneasy. Sitting back in a chair is not a typical sign of potential violence. p. 332, Objective 7

8. False. All patients who are displaying behavioral emergencies should be evaluated to determine if the cause of their problem is medical, trauma, or psychological. p. 333, Objective 6

9. True. Do not argue with a patient who is displaying irrational thinking but do not agree with the patient's disturbed thinking. p. 333, Objectives 6, 8

10. Patients who do not calm down or are showing signs of destructive behavior may need to be *restrained*. p. 334

11. Restraints may help you provide adequate care to the patient, but if used incorrectly they can cause *injury or harm to the patient*. p. 334

12. False. Restraints should be removed by the staff at the receiving facility. If a restraint appears to be too tight, loosen but do not remove the restraint. p. 335

13. False. Patients who are not able to make competent, reasonable decisions can be transported against their will, after consulting medical direc-

tion, local law enforcement, or following local protocols. p. 335, Objective 5

14. When documenting caring for a patient with a behavioral emergency, be sure to include: the position in which the patient was found; any aggressive or abnormal actions by the patient; anything unusual the patient says; aspects of assessment and the findings in detail; restraining procedures used and assessment findings before and after their use; and any persons assisting or witnessing the treatment and transport of the patient. p. 336, Objective 5

15. Assistance in determining the need for transport of a patient refusing care should be obtained through *medical direction*. p. 336, Objective 5

16. The amount of force required to keep patients from injuring themselves or others is called *reasonable force*. p. 336

17. **a.** Assess how the patient actually feels and if the patient expresses suicidal tendencies. Questions to ask this patient include: "What is your name, the date, and your address?", "How do you feel?", "Would you like some help with your problem?", and "Do you have history of diabetes or other medical problem that requires medication?" p. 333. **b.** Ask all questions in a calm and reassuring manner; do not be judgmental; repeat the patient's answers to show that you are listening; always acknowledge how the patient feels; and do not challenge or argue with the patient. p. 334. **c.** Document the position in which the patient was found; any aggressive or abnormal actions; unusual statements; aspects of assessment and findings; any restraining procedures used and assessment and findings before and after their use; and persons assisting or witnessing the treatment and transport. p. 336

● CHAPTER 24
OBSTETRICS AND GYNECOLOGY

● MATCHING

1. O
2. E
3. D
4. K
5. B
6. S
7. I
8. L
9. G
10. M
11. P
12. N
13. J
14. F

15. Q
16. H
17. A
18. R
19. C

Definitions to key terms can be found on page 342 of the student textbook. Key terms cover Objective 1.

● REVIEW QUESTIONS

1. The fetus grows and develops in the *uterus*. p. 352, Objective 1

2. During pregnancy the fetus receives nutrition from the mother through the *placenta*. p. 343, Objective 1

3. False. The placenta is an organ that develops during pregnancy and is expelled from the woman's body after the birth of the baby. p. 343, Objective 1

4. C. There are 1 to 2 L of amniotic fluid in the amniotic sac, surrounding and cushioning the fetus. p. 345, Objective 1

5. B. The usual length of pregnancy is 40 weeks, or approximately 9 months. p. 345

6. During pregnancy a woman's blood volume *increases* to accommodate for the needs of the baby. p. 345

7. True. The first stage of labor begins with the first contractions and ends when the fetus enters the birth canal. The second stage of labor begins when the fetus enters the birth canal and ends when the baby is delivered. The third stage of labor begins with the delivery of the baby and ends with the delivery of the placenta. p. 345

8. False. Crowning is a sign that delivery is very close. If crowning is seen in the assessment of the mother, there is no time to transport the mother and delivery will occur on scene. p. 345, Objective 4

9. The OB kit contains: 1) surgical scissors or a scalpel used to cut the umbilical cord; 2) hemostats or cord clamps used to clamp the umbilical cord; 3) umbilical tape or sterilized cord used to tie the umbilical cord; 4) bulb syringe used to suction the infant's mouth and nose; 5) towels to dry the infant; 6) 2 x 10 gauze sponges to wipe the infant's mouth and nose; 7) sterile gloves to wear during delivery; 8) baby blanket to warm the infant; 9) sanitary napkins for the mother after delivery; and 10) a plastic bag to transport the placenta to the hospital p. 346, Objective 2

10. True. Pregnant women should be treated based on their signs and symptoms, as any other patient would be. The care that is best for the mother will also provide the best care for the fetus. p. 346, Objective 5

11. Labor pains are associated with the contraction of the *uterus*. p. 346, Objective 1

12. False. Labor and delivery involve a large amount of blood and body fluids, so EMT–Basics will need

to wear gloves, eye protection, mask, and gown. p. 356, Objective 7

13. A miscarriage usually occurs in the first 3 months of a pregnancy. p. 346, Objective 3

14. When deciding whether to transport the mother or to assist in delivery on scene, consider: When is the baby due?; Are there any contractions or pain?; Is there any bleeding or discharge?; Is the mother feeling an increasing pressure in the vaginal area?; Does the mother feel the urge to push? Also assess if there is crowning during contractions, and place a gloved hand on the abdomen above the navel to assess contractions. p. 349, Objective 4

15. Have the mother lie on her back with her legs flexed and widely separated. Create a sterile field around the vaginal opening with towels or paper barriers, and place towels across her thighs and abdomen. p. 349, Objective 6

16. B. Gentle pressure should be applied to the perineum, over the baby's head, to prevent an explosive delivery. p. 350, Objectives 8, 9

17. A. Check to ensure that the umbilical cord is not around the baby's neck. If the cord is around the neck, either loosen the cord and slip it over the baby's head or clamp and cut the cord. p. 350, Objectives 8, 9

18. Suction the baby's mouth and nose with the *bulb syringe* prior to the delivery of the torso. p. 350, Objectives 8, 9

19. A. The umbilical cord should be cut between the umbilical clamps after pulsations have stopped in the cord. The first clamp is placed approximately four finger widths away from the baby and the second several inches further from the first clamp. p. 351, Objective 10

20. False. The placenta should be allowed to deliver on its own; never pull on the umbilical cord to pull out the placenta. p. 351, Objective 11

21. False. The placenta must be transported along with the mother and baby to the receiving facility, where it will be evaluated for completeness. p. 351, Objective 11

22. If the mother loses more than 500 mL of blood during the delivery, the EMT–Basic should provide *uterine massage*. If the mother continues to bleed excessively, the uterus should be massaged with both hands fully extended on the lower abdomen above the pubis, which should lessen bleeding. Treat the mother for the signs and symptoms shock, if necessary. p. 354, Objective 12

23. B. The infant is assessed based on appearance, pulse, grimace, activity, and respiratory effort. p. 354

24. The heart rate of a newborn should be greater than *100* beats per minute. p. 355

25. C. If the heart rate is less than 80 beats per minute after ventilations, the EMT–Basic should start chest compressions following neonatal CPR standards. p. 355, Objective 13

26. B. Transport the mother with a prolapsed cord in whatever position will relieve the most pressure from the cord, either with her hips elevated or with her head lowered. p. 357, Objective 14

27. A. Use a gloved hand to make a "V" around the baby's face to prevent suffocation with a breech presentation. p. 357, Objective 14

28. A. Babies from multiple births are often smaller and born earlier than single births. The infants may need to be treated as premature infants are. The mother may not know she is having more than one baby, even if she has had prenatal care. Complication rates are higher for twins, so be prepared with extra personnel. Cut the umbilical cord of the first infant born then prepare for the delivery of the second infant. p. 358, Objective 15

29. True. When one limb presents, the baby cannot deliver in this position and will require a surgical delivery. p. 358, Objective 14

30. True. Meconium, or fetal stool, is usually associated with fetal distress and can create an airway problem. p. 359, Objective 16

31. Infants born at less than 28 weeks, or 7 months, are considered to be *premature*. p. 359, Objective 17

32. True. Premature infants have less developed respiratory and cardiac systems and may require resuscitation. p. 359, Objective 17

33. True. Discourage the patient from washing, bathing, or going to the bathroom until she has been examined and evidence collected. p. 360, Objective 18

34. a. When is the baby due? Are there any contractions or pain? Is there any bleeding or discharge? Is the mother feeling increasing pressure in the vaginal area? Does the mother feel the urge to push? Is there crowning during contractions? p. 349. b. Attempt to loosen the cord and slip it over the baby's head. If the cord cannot be removed, clamp the cord in two places, cut the cord between the two clamps, and remove the cord from the baby's neck. p. 350. c. Record the time of delivery. Transport the mother, infant, and placenta to the hospital. Be sure to keep the infant warm. p. 354

35. a. Provide positive-pressure ventilations at 60/minute with a BVM. p. 355. b. Evaluate the infant's heart rate. If the rate is less than 80/minute and the newborn is not responding to ventilations, start chest compressions. p. 355. c. If the heart rate is above 100/minute and respirations are adequate, administer free-flow oxygen and initiate transport of the mother and infants for physician evaluation. p. 355

1. B. EMT–Basics carry activated charcoal, oral glucose, and oxygen on the EMS unit. EMT–Basics can assist patients with their own physician-prescribed nitroglycerin, epinephrine autoinjectors, and inhalers. p. 237, Objectives 1, 3

2. B. The generic name is listed in the *U.S. Pharmacopeia*, which is a government publication listing all medications used in the United States. The chemical name is a precise description of the chemical composition of the drug. The trade name is assigned by the manufacturer to market the drug. p. 237, Objective 2

3. B. A contraindication is a situation in which a medication should not be used. The medication will not be helpful to the patient and may be harmful. An indication is a common use of a medication for treating an illness or condition. p. 239

4. C. Activated charcoal is a suspension and must be shaken thoroughly to keep the contents mixed. p. 238, Objective 5

5. C. Oral medications have a slow onset of action because they must be absorbed in the digestive system. Oral medications should not be given to unresponsive patients because they will be unable to swallow the medication. Oral medications are a good route of administration for responsive cooperative children. A medication sprayed under the tongue is being administered by the sublingual route. p. 240, Objective 5

6. A. Knowing the side effects of a drug can help the EMT–Basic anticipate their onset and be prepared to deal with any complications. Side effects are the undesirable actions of a drug. The mechanism of action describes how a drug affects the body. EMT–Basics should not help a patient with any medication unless it is approved by medical direction and the EMT–Basic is thoroughly familiar with the drug. p. 241

7. D. The larynx is also known as the voice box. The oropharynx is the part of the throat behind the mouth. The diaphragm is the dome-shaped muscle that separates the thoracic cavity from the abdominal cavity and is used in breathing. The trachea is the windpipe. p. 246, Objective 1

8. C. Respiratory disease can change the shape of a patient's chest over time. Stridor indicates an upper airway obstruction; gurgling is heard when there is liquid in the back of the airway. Agonal respirations are sudden short breaths with long pauses in between, often occurring when the patient is near death. These respirations are not normal in any patient. If a patient is showing signs of hypoxia, the patient should receive high-concentration oxygen, even if the patient normally receives low-concentration oxygen. p. 250, Objectives 2, 3, 5

9. D. A rate of 12 to 20 breaths per minute is normal for an adult patient. Shortness of breath and retractions indicate difficulty breathing in any age group. Other signs of adequate breathing include equal chest expansion, a regular rhythm, and an adequate tidal volume. p. 248

10. B. Proventil and Ventolin are both examples of trade names for albuterol. A medication can have more than one trade name if it is marketed by different manufacturers. p. 253, Objective 8

11. C. To assist a patient with a prescribed inhaler, the patient must have signs and symptoms of respiratory distress and his/her own prescribed inhaler and medical direction must authorize its use. If the patient is unresponsive, the use of an inhaler is contraindicated. EMT–Basics do not carry inhalers on the EMS unit, so the patients must have their own inhaler. p. 254, Objective 5

12. C. Common side effects of a prescribed inhaler use include increased pulse rate, tremors, nervousness, and sometimes nausea. p. 254, Objective 8

13. B. The right ventricle receives oxygen poor blood from the right atrium and then pumps the blood to the lungs via the pulmonary arteries to become saturated with oxygen. The blood then goes to the left atrium, the left ventricle, and the body through the aorta. p. 260, Objective 1

14. D. The signs and symptoms of shock (hypoperfusion) include: a rapid and weak pulse; pale or cyanotic skin; cool, clammy skin; rapid and shallow breathing; restlessness and anxiety; mental dullness; nausea and vomiting; thirst; low blood pressure; and a low temperature. p. 263, Objective 1

15. D. Position responsive patients with no suspected trauma in a position of comfort. Patients experiencing chest pain or difficulty breathing usually prefer sitting up versus lying flat on their back. p. 265, Objectives 2, 7

16. B. Indications for the use of nitroglycerin or conditions that must be met before nitroglycerin is used include signs and symptoms of cardiac chest pain; the patient has his/her own nitroglycerin; and medical direction authorizes its use. Nitroglycerin should not be used if the patient has already taken the maximum dose, if the patient is not mentally alert, or if the blood pressure is less than 100 systolic. p. 266, Objectives 41, 42

17. A. AEDs can be used for patients who weigh more than 41 kg (90 lbs) and who are older than 12 years of age. The patient must be unresponsive and have no pulse for the AED to be applied. p. 270, Objectives 4, 6, 18

18. B. Perform CPR for 1 minute after the first set of three stacked shocks. After 1 minute, reanalyze the patient's rhythm and shock again if the AED indicates this is necessary. p. 273, Objective 25

19. B. Signs and symptoms of a diabetic emergency include an appearance of intoxication, altered mental status, fast heart rate, cool and clammy skin, combativeness, and hunger. p. 285, Objective 1

20. B. Common medication names for the control of diabetes include Humulin, Diabinese, Orinase, and Micronase. Ventolin is a respiratory medication, Dilantin is for seizure control, and Procardia is a cardiac medication. p. 285, Objective 1

21. B. Common causes of seizures include fever, infection, poisoning, intoxication, hypoglycemia, head trauma, hypoxia, and epilepsy. p. 285

22. C. To administer oral glucose, the patient must be alert enough to swallow, have signs and symptoms of altered mental status, and have a known history of diabetes. Oral glucose cannot be administered if the patient is unresponsive or has no known medical history. p. 288, Objectives 2, 4, 5

23. D. Glucose should never be given to an unresponsive patient. Any substance placed in the mouth of an unresponsive patient can cause airway compromise. p. 289, Objectives 3, 4

24. D. An allergic reaction is an exaggerated immune response to an allergen. Common allergens include food (peanuts, shrimp), medications (penicillin, aspirin), plants (poison ivy), and environmental factors (dust, pollen). p. 294, Objective 1

25. B. The SAMPLE history is assessed during the focused history and physical examination for the medical patient. The assessment should be focused on the patient's chief complaint. p. 296, Objective 2

26. B. The adult autoinjector contains 0.3 mg of epinephrine. The child autoinjector generally contains half of the adult dose. p. 197, Objective 5

27. C. The autoinjector is placed against the lateral thigh, midway between the waist and knee. Hold the injector firmly in place until the injector activates. Leave the needle in place for at least 10 seconds. p. 298, Objective 5

28. C. The autoinjector has a sharp needle that has been in direct contact with the patient's body fluid. Dispose of the entire autoinjector in a biohazard container designed for sharps. p. 198

29. A. Common side effects of epinephrine include increased heart rate, pale skin, dizziness, nausea and vomiting, excitability, and anxiousness. p. 198, Objective 5

30. C. When questioning a patient who has overdosed or was poisoned, ask the following questions: "When did you ingest or become exposed to the substance?"; "How much poison did you ingest?"; "Over what time period did the poisoning occur?"; "What has happened since the poisoning?"; "How much do you weigh?" Do not question the patient's motives or accuse the patient of intentional overdose. Cases of suspected negligence or child abuse should be reported to the proper authorities, after the call is over. p. 305, Objective 3

31. B. Ingested toxins often cause nausea, vomiting or diarrhea, altered mental status, abdominal pain, chemical burns around the mouth, and particular breath odors. p. 305, Objectives 1, 2

32. D. Activated charcoal binds to toxins in the patient's stomach. Therefore, it is only useful for patients who have ingested the toxin. p. 311, Objective 6

33. B. The usual dose of activated charcoal for both adult and child patients is 1 g of activated charcoal per kilogram of body weight. p. 311, Objective 6

34. B. Common side effects of activated charcoal include vomiting and black stools. Be prepared to suction if the patient vomits. Medical direction may order the administration of a second dose of activated charcoal if the patient vomits. p. 311, Objective 6

35. C. The body loses heat by conduction (direct transfer of heat), convection (through moving air or liquids), evaporation (when a liquid changes to a gas), radiation (infrared energy), and respiration (exhaling warm air). Shivering raises the body temperature. p. 317, Objective 1

36. C. The skin should be evaluated on the patient's trunk, abdomen, or back. The skin of the extremities is unreliable because blood flow is normally decreased to the extremities to conserve heat. Skin on exposed areas like the face and hands is also unreliable. p. 318, Objective 2

37. A. Signs and symptoms of early generalized hypothermia include rapid pulse; normal blood pressure; rapid breathing; red skin; and reactive pupils. Late signs and symptoms include slow, barely palpable, or irregular pulse; low or absent blood pressure; shallow or absent breathing; pale, cyanotic, or stiff skin; and sluggish pupils. p. 319, Objective 2

38. C. Hot skin, whether moist or dry, indicates the body no longer has the ability to lose heat. This is a sign of an emergency, and the patient should be cooled as quickly as possible. p. 323, Objective 4

39. B. The incidence of spinal injuries is high in water-related emergencies, so be prepared to immobilize the patient if there is an indication of trauma. Drowning means that the patient has died following an immersion incident, near drowning means the patient has survived. Gastric distention should only be relieved if it interferes with ventilation. Immersion in cold water increases the likelihood of resuscitation after long immersion. p. 324, Objectives 5, 6

40. C. Use the edge of a card to scrape the stinger out of the skin. Tweezers may squeeze the venom out of the venom sac. Use of your finger may expose you to the poison or venom. The stinger should be removed so there is no further exposure. p. 325, Objective 8

41. D. Patients considered to be at risk for suicide include patients who: are more than 40 years of

age, are widowed or divorced, are alcoholic, are depressed; have spoken of taking their own lives; have a history of self-destructive behavior; have recently been diagnosed with a serious illness; live in an environment where there is an unusual gathering of destructive articles; have recently lost a loved one; were recently imprisoned; and have recently lost their job. p. 331, Objective 4

42. A. To calm a patient, be sure to tell the patient what you are doing and answer honestly any questions the patient may have. Repeat the patient's answers to your questions to show you are listening. Do not be judgmental toward the patient. Include family members and friends in your assessment of the patient. p. 334, Objective 8

43. C. EMT–Basics should use wide, soft restraints to avoid cutting off distal circulation to an extremity. Behavioral emergency patients should be assessed for illness or injury. Ask patients about their past medical history to search for clues relating to their behavioral emergency. Same-sex attendants should be used whenever possible, and EMT–Basics should have witnesses with them when caring for a patient with a behavioral emergency. p. 335, Objective 5

44. C. When restraining a patient, use only the amount of force necessary to keep the patient from injuring him/herself or others. This is known as reasonable force. p. 336, Objectives 6

45. B. The uterus is the organ in which a growing fetus develops. The uterus contracts during labor to push the baby out of the birth canal. The amniotic sac surrounds the fetus with 1 to 2 L of amniotic fluid and helps cushion the fetus from injury. The birth canal is the lower part of the uterus and the vagina. The perineum is the area of skin between the vagina and anus. p. 343, Objective 1

46. A. The first stage of labor begins with regular contractions of the uterus and ends when the baby enters the birth canal. The second stage of labor begins with the baby entering the birth canal and ends when the baby is delivered. The third stage of labor begins when the baby is delivered and ends when the placenta is delivered. p. 345, Objective 4

47. C. Magill forceps are not usually found in the obstetrical kit. The OB kit routinely contains surgical scissors or a scalpel, hemostats or cord clamps, umbilical tape or sterilized cord, a bulb syringe, towels, 2 x 10 gauze sponges, sterile gloves, a baby blanket, sanitary napkins, and a plastic bag. p. 346, Objective 2

48. B. The mother should not be allowed to use the toilet because the baby may deliver while she is trying to have a bowel movement. If contractions are less than 2 minutes apart, the mother feels a strong need to push, or if the baby is crowning, prepare for delivery on scene. p. 349, Objectives 4, 6

49. B. The umbilical cord should be cut approximately 4 finger widths from the baby after being clamped. p. 352, Objective 10

50. C. Uterine massage will help slow bleeding. Losing up to 500 cc of blood is normal for delivery. p. 354, Objective 12

51. B. Prolapsed cord is when the umbilical cord is the presenting part. Breech delivery means the buttocks or both legs deliver first. Meconium is fetal stool that may be present in the amniotic fluid, indicating fetal distress. p. 359, Objective 14

● CHAPTER 25 BLEEDING AND SHOCK

● MATCHING

1. A
2. G
3. E
4. H
5. C
6. D
7. I
8. F
9. B

Definitions to key terms can be found on page 367 of the student textbook.

● REVIEW QUESTIONS

1. The cardiovascular system delivers *blood* through a system of *arteries, veins,* and capillaries. p. 368, Objective 1

2. C. The average adult has approximately 6 L of blood in the body. p. 368, Objective 1

3. False. Not every part of the body needs to be perfused equally at all times. For example, the muscles in your thighs require more blood flow when you are jogging than when you are lying down. p. 369, Objective 1

4. A. The systolic pressure is a measure of the pressure against the arteries when the heart contracts; the diastolic pressure is a measure of the pressure against the arteries when the heart is at rest. p. 369, Objective 1

5. Good perfusion of the body requires an adequate *blood pressure.* p. 369, Objective 1

6. A decrease in perfusion to the cells in the body results in hypoperfusion or *shock.* p. 369, Objective 1

7. When tissues are not adequately perfused they are damaged by lack of *oxygen* and a build-up of *waste products.* p. 369, Objective 9

8. The four major organs easily damaged by hypoperfusion are the brain, heart, lungs, and kidneys. p. 369, Objective 1

9. Some of the causes of hypovolemic shock include: dehydration; vomiting; diarrhea; internal blood loss; and external blood loss. p. 370, Objective 1

10. B. Changes in mental status are some of the most sensitive indicators or hypoperfusion. These mental status changes can include restlessness, anxiety, or combativeness. p. 370, Objective 9

11. False. Vasoconstriction means that the blood vessels constrict, allowing less blood to be delivered to an area of the body. Because less blood is directed toward an area, the skin becomes pale, cool, and clammy. p. 370, Objective 9

12. True. As the body tries to adjust for lowering blood pressures, less blood is directed toward the nonessential areas of the body, such as the extremities, so that more blood can be directed toward the heart, lungs, and brain. Less blood flow means that there will be weaker pulses. p. 370, Objective 9

13. B. Capillary refill should return the pink color to the skin in less than 2 seconds in adequately perfusing patients. Capillary refill is only measured in children less than 6 years of age. p. 371, Objective 9

14. C. The heart rate will increase to try to meet the body's demands for more oxygen. p. 371, Objective 9

15. A late sign of shock is a *decreased* blood pressure. p. 371, Objective 9

16. The first priority with any patient is to ensure an *open airway*. p. 372, Objective 5

17. The legs can be elevated to place a patient in the shock position, as long as there are no injuries or suspected injuries to the: a) spine, c) pelvis, d) lower extremities, e) head, f) chest, or g) abdomen. Lifting the legs would aggravate an injury to any of these areas of the body. p. 373, Objective 10

18. True. Always practice proper body substance isolation precautions when there is external trauma. p. 374, Objective 4

19. A sudden loss of 1 L of blood for an adult patient is considered to be a serious blood loss. p. 374, Objective 1

20. C. Blood coming from an artery is under high pressure and will spurt with each heartbeat. p. 374, Objective 2

21. D. Blood coming from a vein is under lower pressure than blood from an artery and will flow from the injury site. p. 375, Objective 2

22. Bleeding from capillaries is usually minimal and will ooze from the injury site. p. 375, Objective 2

23. B. Concentrated direct pressure will put the maximum amount of pressure on the isolated injury site. p. 375, Objective 3

24. When there is no one isolated point of bleeding, diffuse direct pressure is the best method to control bleeding. Pressure points, extremity elevation, and splinting will also be effective in controlling bleeding. p. 375, Objective 3

25. *Elevating* an injury above the level of the heart may help decrease blood flow to that area, and therefore decrease bleeding. An extremity cannot be elevated if it is injured. p. 376, Objective 3

26. C. By placing pressure against a pressure point, you can minimize the amount of blood flowing to the injury site. Because most areas of the body are perfused by more than one artery, this will slow bleeding but not stop it entirely. p. 376, Objective 3

27. True. Splinting an injury will help minimize bleeding by reducing the motion of sharp bone ends. p. 377, Objective 3

28. True. Using PASG when a patient has a chest injury may make it more difficult for the patient to breathe and cause respiratory compromise. p. 378, Objective 8

29. The last resort for bleeding control is applying a *tourniquet*. p. 379, Objective 3

30. B. Tourniquets should not be removed once they are applied, because a blood clot could be released into the circulation. p. 380, Objective 3

31. If a tourniquet is used, always avoid placing it over a *joint* injury. p. 380, Objective 3

32. Bleeding from the ears and nose can be a sign of a *skull fracture* in a trauma patient. p. 381, Objective 7

33. False. It is difficult to apply direct pressure to the site of bleeding from the ears and nose. For nose bleeds, pinch the fleshy part of the nostrils together. p. 381, Objective 8

34. If a patient has signs and symptoms of shock (hypoperfusion) and a serious mechanism of injury with no obvious bleeding, you should suspect *internal bleeding*. p. 383, Objectives 6, 7

35. Signs and symptoms of internal bleeding include: signs and symptoms of shock; bleeding from any body orifice; blood-tinged vomit or feces; coffee-ground vomit; dark tarry stool; abdominal rigidity or tenderness; and distended abdomen. p. 383, Objective 7

36. If you suspect a patient is bleeding internally, you would follow BSI precautions, maintain an open airway and adequate ventilation, treat the patient for the signs and symptoms of shock, splint the injured femur, apply the PASG (if indicated), and transport immediately. p. 384, Objective 8

37. The PASG may be considered if the patient has signs and symptoms of shock, a tender abdomen, and suspected pelvic injury. The PASG should not be used if the patient has a chest injury. Local protocol and the presence or absence of other injuries will determine if the PASG is used. p. 383, Objective 8

38. a. High-concentration oxygen will decrease cell death from the hypoxia caused by hypoperfusion. p. 373. b. The next steps to use in controlling bleeding are extremity elevation and pressure points. Because the patient has an open injury to this lower extremity, elevation would be not be

appropriate. Attempt to control the bleeding by applying pressure to the patient's femoral artery. p. 376. **c.** The PASG is helpful for immobilizing injuries to the lower extremity and in controlling bleeding in the lower extremities. p. 377

39. **a.** Bright-red bloody stools indicate bleeding in the lower gastrointestinal tract. p. 383. **b.** A lowered blood pressure, an increased pulse rate, and increased respirations are classic signs of hypoperfusion due to hypovolemia. p. 371. **c.** To treat this patient use appropriate BSI precautions, maintain an open airway, provide 100% oxygen, elevate the patent's legs 8 to 12 inches, prevent heat loss, and transport immediately. p. 373

● CHAPTER 26
SOFT-TISSUE INJURIES

● MATCHING

1. A
2. J
3. D
4. F
5. M
6. C
7. B
8. E
9. I
10. O
11. H
12. N
13. L
14. K
15. G

Definitions to key terms can be found on page 389 of the student textbook. Key terms cover Objectives 4, 6, 11, 12, 14, 16, 21, and 22.

● REVIEW QUESTIONS

1. The skin serves as a barrier from infection, regulates body temperature, and contains nerve endings to transmit information to the brain. p. 390, Objective 1

2. B. Nerve endings are found in the dermis, along with sweat and sebaceous glands, hair follicles, and small blood vessels. p. 390, Objective 2

3. A closed injury is defined as an injury in which the skin remains intact and there is no external bleeding. p. 392, Objective 4

4. A. A contusion or bruise is discoloration of the skin caused by trauma. p. 392, Objective 4

5. B. A hematoma is a large collection of blood under the skin, producing pain and discoloration. p. 392, Objective 4

6. An open injury occurs when the skin is broken and there is external bleeding. p. 392, Objective 6

7. B. Abrasions occur when the outermost layers of the skin are scraped away. p. 392, Objective 6

8. C. Lacerations can be regular or irregular and are caused when an object tears the skin. p. 393, Objective 6

9. A. Gunshot and stab wounds are examples of penetrations and punctures. p. 393, Objective 6

10. D. An amputation occurs when an appendage, such as a finger or toe, is removed from the body. p. 394, Objective 6

11. True. Soft-tissue injuries are often bloody, and the EMT–Basic will need to take proper body substance isolation precautions. p. 394, Objective 3

12. False. An appropriately sized dressing should cover the wound with about 1 inch to spare on all sides. p. 395, Objective 7

13. Pressure can be applied by applying a bandage tightly to an injury, using gauze rolls to wrap around the injury, or using an air splint. p. 395, Objective 23

14. An occlusive dressing taped on *three* sides allows air to *escape* but not *enter* the wound. p. 397, Objectives 7, 8, 10

15. False. Eviscerated abdominal contents should be protected with a moist, sterile dressing to prevent the contents from drying out. p. 397, Objectives 9, 10

16. Impaled objects should be removed when they are in the cheek and causing airway compromise, when they interfere with CPR, or when the patient cannot be transported because of the object. p. 397, Objective 26

17. B. Because both eyes move together, both eyes should be covered to minimize movement of the injured eye. p. 397, Objectives 5, 7

18. False. Amputated parts should be placed in a sterile dressing and then wrapped in plastic. Keep the part cool, but not frozen. p. 397, Objective 27

19. The priority for care for all patients is to manage the *airway*. Caring for bleeding, amputations, eviscerations, and burns are all secondary to maintaining a patent airway.

20. B. Immobilize a partial amputation to prevent it from becoming a complete amputation. Dress and bandage the injury to minimize bleeding and contamination. p. 399, Objective 27

21. Direct pressure can be used on the head only if there is no evidence of a *skull fracture*. p. 399, Objective 5

22. B. When the patient has injuries involving the mouth, evaluate for the presence of blood and teeth, which may create an airway compromise. p. 400, Objective 7

23. To determine the severity of a burn, evaluate the depth of the burn, the total percentage of body surface area burned, the location of the burn, any

preexisting medical conditions, and the age of the patient. p. 400, Objective 11

24. A sunburn is a type of *superficial* burn. p. 400, Objectives 12, 13

25. Dry, leathery, charred skin with little or no pain describes a *full-thickness* burn. p. 400, Objectives 16, 17

26. If blisters form, the burn is considered to be *partial thickness*. p. 400, Objectives 14, 15

27. In the "Rule of Nines" the head of an adult is *9%* of the total body surface area and the head of an infant is *18%*. p. 402 , Objective 11

28. True. A circumferential burn of the torso can cause swelling and inhibit the chest rise, causing respiratory compromise. p. 401

29. Five critical areas for burns are the face, upper airway, hands, feet, and genitalia. p. 401

30. c—partial-thickness burn of the face; mod—child with a partial-thickness burn of less than 10%; mod—full-thickness burn of less than 2%; min—partial-thickness burn covering 27% of the body. A partial-thickness burn of the face would be a critical burn. A child with a partial-thickness burn of less than 10% and a full-thickness burn of less than 2% are both minor burns. A partial-thickness burn of 27% of the body is a moderate burn. p. 403, Objective 11

31. A. Burned patients are at risk for hypothermia and infection because the skin has been damaged. These patients must be kept warm. p. 403, Objectives 18, 19, 20

32. True. Jewelry and clothing must be removed when treating a burn patient, because the burned area is likely to swell and these items could be constricting. p. 403, Objectives 18, 19, 20

33. If a patient has suffered a chemical burn from dry powder, first *brush off* the powder then *flush* with water. p. 403, Objective 28

34. When treating a patient with *electrical* burns, be prepared with the AED because cardiac arrest is more likely. Ensure that the patient is no longer in contact with the electrical source before beginning treatment. p. 404, Objective 29

35. a. To treat soft-tissue injuries, you should: ensure a patent airway and provide ventilatory support as needed; if the patient is showing signs and symptoms of shock, administer high-flow oxygen via a nonrebreather mask; expose the wound, control the bleeding, and minimize contamination with a dry sterile dressing; assess for possible spine injury; and splint extremity injuries. p. 394. b. If the dressing becomes saturated, remove the dressing and apply fingertip pressure (with a gloved hand) directly at the site. p. 395. c. If the patient has signs and symptoms of shock, administer high-flow oxygen via a nonrebreather mask at 15 L/min; place the patient in a supine position;

transport the patient as soon as possible; and try to keep the patient calm and quiet. p. 394

36. a. A partial-thickness burn involves both the epidermis and dermis but not the underlying tissue. A full-thickness burn extends through all layers of the skin to the underlying tissue, including the subcutaneous layer, and may involve the muscle, bone, or other organs. p. 400. b. 45%. Anterior chest and abdomen (18%), right arm (9%), right leg (18%). p. 402. c. When caring for burn patients, use BSI precautions; use room-temperature water or saline to cool the burn; remove jewelry and smoldering clothes; continually monitor the airway; apply high-flow oxygen; cover the burns with dry, clean dressings; and keep the patient warm during transport to the nearest burn facility according to protocol. p. 403

● CHAPTER 27
MUSCULOSKELETAL CARE

● MATCHING

1. J
2. I
3. E
4. A
5. B
6. F
7. D
8. K
9. M
10. C
11. G
12. H
13. L

Definitions to key terms can be found on page 409 of the student textbook.

● REVIEW QUESTIONS

1. Muscles give shape to the body, protect internal organs, and provide for movement of the body. p. 410, Objective 1

2. Skeletal muscles are attached to *bones* and are responsible for *movement*. p. 410, Objective 1

3. Muscles over which we have no direct control are called *involuntary* or *smooth* muscle. p. 410, Objective 1

4. Automaticity is a characteristic found only in *cardiac* muscle. Automaticity means that the muscle can contract on its own. Voluntary and involuntary muscles must receive an impulse from the brain to contract or relax. p. 411, Objective 1

5. a. Vertebral; b. Scapula; c. Radius; d. Ulna; e. Clavicle; f. Sternum; g. Humerus; h. Femur; i. Patella; j. Tibia; k. Fibula. p. 64, Objective 3

6. **a.** Cervical vertebrae; **b.** Thoracic vertebrae; **c.** Lumbar; **d.** Sacral vertebrae; **e.** Fused coccyx. p. 65, Objective 3

7. The skeletal system gives shape to the body, protects internal organs, and provides for movement of the body. p. 411, Objective 2

8. The knee is an example of a *hinge* joint, and a hip is a *ball and socket* joint. p. 411, Objective 2

9. **a.** fist to the jaw; **c.** internal organs against the chest in an automobile crash; **b.** running back tackled after turning from a catch. p. 412

10. Signs and symptoms of a musculoskeletal injury include: deformity or angulation; pain and tenderness; crepitation; swelling; bruising; exposed bone ends; and joints locked into position. p. 413, Objective 4

11. True. Splinting is performed after the assessment of airway, breathing, and circulation is complete and no immediate threats to life are found. p. 413, Objectives 6, 8

12. Splinting *minimizes* the amount of movement of sharp bone ends, and therefore *minimizes* damage to surrounding muscles and nerves. Splinting also reduces pain for the patient. p. 414, Objective 5

13. Pulse, motor function, and sensation must be evaluated *before* and *after* splinting. p. 414, Objective 6

14. If the distal pulse changes after splinting, *loosen* the splint and reassess. p. 414, Objective 6

15. False. The position of function is the most natural position for the hand or foot, where the least muscle is stretched. The position of function for the hand is with the palms bent and fingers slightly curled. p. 415, Objective 6

16. To be effective, the splint must include the joint *above* and *below* a long bone injury. p. 415, Objective 6

17. Full body immobilization should be used if *spinal* trauma is suspected. p. 415, Objective 8

18. B. Traction splints are used only on midshaft femur injuries, with no involvement of the hip, knee, or lower leg. p. 415, Objective 8

19. Pneumatic splints are good for *angulated* injuries because they allow the extremity to remain in the position found. p. 416, Objective 8

20. Pneumatic splints apply pressure to sites of bleeding, provide uniform contact for the extremity, and are comfortable for the patient. p. 416, Objective 8

21. True. The PASG can be used to immobilize suspected injuries to the pelvis and femur. p. 417, Objective 8

22. Shoulder injuries usually require a *sling and swathe* for stabilization. p. 419, Objective 8

23. A splint that is too loose will not keep the extremity immobilized. A splint that is too tight will cut off distal circulation and possibly cause permanent damage. Splints can compress nerves, tissues, and blood vessels. An improperly applied splint can increase bleeding and tissue damage, cause permanent nerve damage or disability, convert a closed injury to an open injury, or increase pain. p. 419, Objective 7

24. **a.** Signs and symptoms of a bone or joint injury include: deformity or angulation; pain and tenderness; crepitation; swelling; bruising; exposed bone ends; and joints locked into position. p. 413. **b.** Evaluate the pulse, motor function, and sensation distal to the injury both before and after applying a splint and record findings. p. 414. **c.** Align the injury with gentle traction before splinting; pad the splint to prevent pressure and discomfort; and immobilize the hand in the position of function by placing a roll of gauze in the palm to support the hand. p. 414

● CHAPTER 28
INJURIES TO THE HEAD AND SPINE

● MATCHING
1. E
2. F
3. A
4. B
5. C
6. D

Definitions to key terms can be found on page 425 of the student textbook.

● REVIEW QUESTIONS
1. The components of the central nervous system are the *brain* and the *spinal cord*. p. 426, Objective 1

2. Cerebral spinal fluid (CSF) surrounds the *brain* and spinal cord and acts as a *cushion*. p. 426, Objective 1

3. Sensory nerves carry information *from* the body *to* the brain. Sensory nerves carry information regarding pressure, pain, heat, etc. from the body to the spinal cord and brain. Motor nerves carry information from the brain to the body. p. 426, Objective 2

4. The spinal column contains *33* bones. p. 426, Objective 3

5. There are seven cervical vertebrae, 12 thoracic vertebrae, five lumbar vertebra, five sacral vertebrae, and four coccygeal vertebrae. p. 427, Objective 3

6. False. Cervical spine immobilization devices do not provide enough immobilization for the patient's head. The EMT–Basic must still provide manual stabilization until the head is immobilized to the long backboard. p. 430, Objective 9

7. A short backboard is used to immobilize the head, neck, and torso when the patient is in the *seated* position. p. 430, Objective 15

8. Long backboards provide *full* body immobilization. p. 430

9. False. The patient's head must be secured to the long backboard with a cervical spine immobilization device or tape, and straps are required to keep the body secured to the board. p. 430, Objective 9

10. Mechanism of injury refers to how the injury occurred and how much force was applied to the patient's body during the incident. p. 430, Objective 4

11. B. Knowing the mechanism of injury allows you to know what types of forces caused the patient's injuries. This may lead you to discover hidden injuries. p. 431, Objective 4

12. Significant mechanisms of injury include: motor vehicle crashes; pedestrians injured in vehicle collisions; falls; blunt trauma to the head, chest, abdomen, or pelvis; penetrating trauma to the head, neck, or torso; motorcycle crashes; hanging; diving accidents; and any trauma that results in an unresponsive patient. p. 431, Objective 4

13. A hanging will cause b) distraction, or pulling apart of the spine. A dive into shallow water will cause a) compression of the head and spinal column. Rear-end automobile crashes will cause the head to jerk backward and then forward, causing c) excessive flexion and extension. p. 431, Objective 4

14. True. Do not ask a patient to move an injured area just to see if there is pain. Immobilize the injured area. p. 432, Objective 7

15. Injuries to the shoulder and chest can cause trauma to the *spine*. Injuries to the lumbar or thoracic vertebrae are more likely if there is injury to the shoulder or chest. p. 432, Objective 6

16. Numbness, tingling, or weakness are possible signs and symptoms of a *spinal injury*. Paralysis also is another sign of a spinal injury. p. 432, Objective 6

17. Ask responsive trauma patients: "What happened?"; "Where does it hurt?"; "Does your neck or back hurt?"; "Can you move your fingers and toes?"; "Where am I touching you now?" p. 433, Objective 6

18. DCAP-BTLS is an acronym for Deformities, Contusions, Abrasions, Penetrations/Punctures, Burns, Tenderness, Lacerations, and Swelling. p. 433

19. After every intervention assess *vital signs, motor function*, and *sensory function*. p. 433, Objective 14

20. True. It is important to document any findings or changes in the patient's condition and to report them to the receiving facility. p. 433

21. It may be helpful to complete the assessment of the cervical region *prior* to applying the cervical spine immobilization device. If you assess after the device is applied, you will need to remove the device. p. 433, Objective 10

22. The patient with spinal cord injury may have difficulty breathing if the nerves that control the diaphragm are injured. EMT–Basics must carefully assess the patient's breathing status and assist with ventilations if indicated. p. 433, Objectives 8, 11

23. A. Cervical spine immobilization devices and complete spinal immobilization are indicated for patients whose mechanism of injury suggests that they may have injured their head, neck, or back. The cervical spine immobilization device needs to be sized appropriately, and the sizing techniques vary with different brands of devices. If moving the patient's head into neutral alignment causes pain, immobilize the head in the position found. Manual stabilization must be maintained until the patient is completely immobilized. p. 434, Objective 12

24. C. The patient's head should be immobilized to the long backboard after the shoulders and hips are secured. The legs and arms can be secured after the head is immobilized. The EMT–Basic at the head of the patient is responsible for calling patient movements. If the patient is not aligned on the long backboard, move the patient either upwards or downwards on the board, never push from side to side. p. 435, Objectives 13, 14

25. 3—secure the torso to the board; 2—place the backboard behind the patient; 7—reassess pulse, motor function, and sensation; 6—secure the arms, legs, and feet; 4—pad the voids behind the patient's head; 1—attach the straps to the board; 5—secure the head to the board; p. 437, Objective 16

26. To immobilize a seated patient you can use a *short backboard* or a *vest type device*. p. 440, Objective 16

27. Patients on short spine boards or KEDs must then be secured to a *long backboard* for transport. p. 440, Objective 16

28. Spinal injuries also may involve injuries to the *brain* and *skull*. p. 440

29. False. Scalp wounds tend to bleed a lot. Bleeding from the scalp usually can be controlled with direct pressure. p. 441

30. The best indicator of a traumatic head injury is *altered mental status*. p. 442

31. Signs and symptoms of head injury include: altered mental status; irregular breathing pattern; mechanism of injury such as deformity of a windshield or helmet; deformity to the skull or a soft area or depression; blood or other fluid leaking from the ears and/or nose; bruising around the eyes or ears; neurologic disability; nausea and/or vomiting; unequal pupil size with altered mental status; seizure activity; contusion, lacerations or hematomas on the scalp; penetrating injury; and exposed brain tissue. p. 442

32. A patient should be rapidly extricated when: 1) the scene is unsafe; 2) the patient's condition is unstable and warrants immediate movement and transport; or 3) when the patient blocks access to another more seriously injured patient. p. 442, Objective 17

33. C. The helmet should not be removed if it will cause further injury. Helmets should be removed when the patient's airway or breathing cannot be controlled with the helmet in place, if the helmet does not fit properly and allows for excessive motion, or if the head cannot be immobilized to the backboard with the helmet in place. p. 444, Objectives 19, 20

34. A. Sports helmets are typically open in the front, making access to the airway simple. Full face shield helmets will not allow the EMT–Basic to assess the airway and generally should be removed. If the helmet is left in place, a cervical spine immobilization device probably will not provide adequate immobilization, and you will need to use tape, towels, and bulky dressings in addition to the device. Shoulder pads will need to be removed if a football helmet is removed to keep the spine in neutral alignment. p. 444, Objectives 21, 22, 26

35. C. The head is immobilized by placing one hand on the mandible at the angle of the jaw and the other hand posteriorly at the occipital region. EMT–Basics should reposition their hands as necessary to prevent the head from falling back. p. 445, Objectives 23, 25

36. For an infant or small child, padding may have to be placed under the *shoulder to heels* to maintain neutral alignment. p. 444

37. True. Osteoporosis and arthritis are two examples of diseases that may make it difficult to immobilize an older patient. p. 447

38. **a.** Airway control with spinal precautions is always the priority. p. 433. **b.** Bleeding of the scalp should be controlled with direct pressure, unless a skull fracture is suspected. p. 441. **c.** Signs and symptoms of head injury include: altered mental status; irregular breathing patterns; deformity to the skull; blood or other fluid leaking from the ears and/or nose; bruising around the eyes and/or behind the ears (this is a late sign, occurring 2-4 hours after injury); neurologic disability; nausea and/or vomiting; and unequal pupil size. p. 442

● DIVISION FIVE EXAMINATION

1. C. Hypovolemic shock occurs when there is an inadequate volume of blood for the heart to pump and circulate. All organs do not need to be perfused equally at all times. The heart, lungs, kidneys and brain, for example, need a continuous supply of blood for the body to function and cannot tolerate an interruption in the supply of blood. The average adult has 5 to 6 L of blood in his/her body. p. 370, Objective 9

2. A. Changes in mental status occur due to changes in the perfusion of the brain. Patients experiencing altered mental status may not be getting an adequate supply of blood to the brain. Changes in mental status are an early indicator of hypoperfusion, occurring much earlier than changes in blood pressure. p. 370, Objective 9

3. D. Signs and symptoms of shock include: restlessness, anxiety, combativeness, increased heart rate, decreased capillary refill in infants and children (greater than 2 seconds), pale or clammy skin, thirst, decreasing level of responsiveness, breathing changes, nausea and vomiting, decreased blood pressure, cyanosis, and sluggishly reactive pupils. p. 372, Objective 9

4. B. When treating a patient with signs and symptoms of shock, maintain an open airway, provide 100% oxygen, control bleeding, elevate the legs and lie the patient down, keep the patient warm, and transport immediately. Low blood pressure in a patient is a sign of late shock, so injuries should be splinted en route to the receiving facility to expedite transport. p. 373, Objectives 9, 10

5. A. Sudden loss of 1 L of blood is considered to be serious in healthy adult patients. Children bleed at the same rate as adults, so equal injuries are more serious for children. Geriatric patients cannot compensate for blood loss as well as a healthy adult patient can. Blood loss of as little as 100 mL is considered to be serious for an infant. p. 374, Objective 3

6. B. Arterial bleeding is bright red, under high pressure and may spurt, and is difficult to control. Venous bleeding is a darker red color, under low pressure, and flows in a steady stream. Capillary bleeding is dark red and usually oozes from the site. p. 375, Objective 2

7. A. If the bleeding is from one main source, concentrated direct pressure applied with your fingertips is preferred to control bleeding. p. 375, Objective 3

8. D. Tourniquets cause extensive tissue damage, sometimes requiring amputation of tissue distal to the tourniquet. For this reason, tourniquets are used as a last resort. When a tourniquet is used, a wide band that will not cut the patient is needed. Tourniquets are rarely required, even in cases of amputation. p. 379, Objective 3

9. D. Signs and symptoms of external bleeding include signs and symptoms of shock, bleeding from any body orifice, blood-tinged vomit or feces, coffee ground vomit, dark tarry stool, abdominal rigidity or tenderness, and a distended abdomen. When caring for epistaxis (nosebleed), have the patient lean forward so he/she does not

swallow blood. Up to 225 mL of blood can be lost in a closed tibia injury. p. 383, Objectives 7, 8

10. A. The outer layer of skin is the epidermis, the middle layer is the dermis, and the tissue underlying the dermis is the subcutaneous layer. p. 391, Objective 2

11. C. An abrasion is a scrape, generally with capillary bleeding. A contusion is a bruise, an avulsion is a flap of skin torn loose, and a crush injury occurs when force is applied with a blunt instrument. p. 392, Objective 6

12. C. A contusion and a hematoma are closed injuries. An abrasion, laceration, avulsion, penetration and puncture are all open injuries. Crush injuries can be open or closed. p. 392, Objective 4

13. D. An avulsion involves a piece of skin that is torn loose or completely off. p. 393, Objective 6

14. C. Extremities that are injured should be splinted, if time allows, to minimize pain and bleeding. Bandages are used to secure dressings in place. An occlusive dressing is nonporous, preventing air from entering a wound. Injuries to joints should be bandaged in the position in which they are found. p. 395, Objective 7

15. A. An evisceration is an abdominal injury in which the abdominal contents are exposed. The EMT–Basic should cover the organs and wound to prevent the contents from drying. p. 397, Objective 9

16. B. Impaled objects in the cheek can be removed if they obstruct the airway. Dress the wound on the inside and outside of the mouth. p. 397, Objective 26

17. B. Amputated body parts should be placed in a plastic bag and kept cool. Do not freeze amputated parts, allow them to become warm, or place them directly on ice or in water. p. 399, Objective 27

18. B. A partial-thickness burn is intensely painful and causes blisters. A superficial burn causes pain and red skin. A full-thickness burn will appear dry and leathery and have little or no pain. p. 400, Objective 15

19. C. Following the Rule of Nines, each leg is 14% body surface and the arm is 9% body surface, totalling 37%. p. 401, Objective 11

20. A. A partial-thickness burn involving the feet, hands, genitalia, or face is considered to be a critical burn. Burns caused by dry lime should not be flushed, because water will react with the lime causing more damage. Electrical burns cause extensive internal damage to the body, with minor damage to the skin. Burn patients cannot regulate their body heat, so they must be kept warm. p. 403, Objective 19

21. C. Involuntary muscle, or smooth muscle, is located in the walls of the hollow structure of the gastrointestinal tract, in the urinary system, in the blood vessels, and in the lungs. Voluntary muscle, or skeletal muscle, attaches to bones to provide for movement. Cardiac muscle is found in the heart and contracts to make the heart beat. p. 411, Objective 1

22. A. A direct injury occurs when a force acts on a body part, such as a baseball bat striking an arm. Indirect injury means the force was applied somewhere on the body, and the injury is in a different place. Twisting force is applied when an extremity is pulled or twisted. p. 412

23. B. Crepitation is the sound heard when bone ends rub together. When there is crepitation, the EMT–Basic may feel grating when palpating the injury. p. 412

24. B. When splinting a joint injury, immobilize the bone above and below the injury. Assess distal pulse, sensation, and motor function before and after splinting. Remove clothing around an injury so that you can examine the injury and so the clothing does not become constricting if the injury swells. Protruding bone ends should not be replaced when splinting an injury. p. 413, Objective 6

25. B. If the patient has signs and symptoms of shock, there is no time to splint each individual extremity. Align the body in the normal anatomic position, and splint the entire body to the long backboard. p. 415, Objective 8

26. A. Traction splints are used for injuries that are isolated to the midfemur. Do not use a traction splint if the injury involves the pelvis, knee, or the lower extremities. p. 415, Objective 6

27. A. The central nervous system is composed of the brain and spinal cord. The peripheral nervous system is composed of motor nerves and sensory nerves. p. 426, Objective 1

28. C. A properly sized cervical spine immobilization device will immobilize the head in the neutral position. The device will not allow the head to move from side to side or up and down excessively. The chin should fit comfortably in the chin rest without slipping out of place. The rescuer holding the head must maintain stabilization until the head is immobilized to the long backboard. p. 429, Objective 10

29. B. If you do not have the proper size cervical spine immobilization device, use rolled towels on either side of the patient's head and tape them in place. Do not use a device that is too small or too large. p. 430, Objective 10

30. D. After immobilizing a patient to a short or long backboard, reassess pulse, motor function, and sensation in the extremities. The head should be secured to the long backboard after the body, and a cervical spine immobilization device should always be used. When using a KED, buckle the lower chest straps before the top chest strap. p. 430, Objectives 14, 16

31. B. Compression injuries of the spine occur when the head is pushed downward and the spine is compressed. Distraction occurs when the spine is pulled apart. Flexion and extension can occur when the head snaps forward and backward. p. 431, Objective 4

32. C. Always reassess pulse, motor function, and sensation after every intervention. Patients who have no pain can still have injuries to the spine. Patients with injuries to their pelvis can have injuries to their lower spine. Manual stabilization of the head should be maintained from the beginning of the initial assessment until the patient is immobilized on the long backboard. p. 430, Objectives 14, 16

33. C. Rapid extrication should be used when there is immediate danger to the EMT–Basic or the patient, when the patient cannot be treated in the position he/she is in, and if life-saving care cannot be provided to another patient unless this patient is moved. If the scene is unsafe for the EMT–Basic to enter, no care should be provided until the scene is made safe. p. 443, Objective 17

34. D. Helmets should be removed if you cannot assess or treat the patient because the helmet is in the way, if the helmet is loose, and if the head cannot be immobilized with the helmet in place. p. 444, Objective 20

35. D. Children have relatively large heads in proportion to the rest of their bodies, requiring special immobilization techniques. Pad the patient from the shoulders to the toes to achieve neutral alignment. Make sure the straps are tight so the child feels secure. Geriatric patients may have conditions that will not allow their spines to be straightened, so apply extra padding for comfort and to immobilize. p. 447, Objective 14

● CHAPTER 29
INFANT AND CHILD EMERGENCY CARE

● MATCHING

1. A
2. N
3. R
4. J
5. O
6. D
7. G
8. S
9. I
10. B
11. K
12. M
13. Q
14. U
15. C
16. H
17. F
18. L
19. E
20. P
21. T

Definitions to key terms can be found on page 455 of the student textbook. Key terms cover Objective 1.

● REVIEW QUESTIONS

1. True. These patients have a large body surface area and have immature thermoregulatory systems. They are also unable to put on or remove clothing by themselves. Be sure to cover the patient or replace the patient's clothing after examination. p. 456, Objectives 1, 2, 3

2. To get the most information about an infant or newborn, assess the *heart and lungs* first and then move to the *head*. If you can assess the heart and lungs, before they get upset, you will obtain more accurate information. p. 457, Objectives 1, 3

3. Evaluate an infant's respirations by watching the effort of breathing; by watching the chest rise and fall; by looking at the infant's skin color, level of activity, and use of accessory muscles to breathe; and by watching the infant's interactions with caregivers. p. 457, Objectives 1, 2, 3

4. False. Most toddlers do not like to be touched by strangers. p. 457, Objectives 1, 3

5. True. Parents can relay vital information about their child and keep them calm during your evaluation. Allow the parent and child to remain together whenever possible. p. 457, Objectives 1, 3

6. Most preschoolers like to *explore* and will often be easily distracted by your equipment. Allow the child to look at and touch equipment before you use it, if time and the patient's condition allow. p. 457, Objectives 1, 3

7. True. School-age children should be able to explain to you the circumstances surrounding an accident or events prior to an illness. p. 457, Objectives 1, 3

8. c—school age; b—adolescent; d—infant; a—toddler. p. 458, Objectives 1, 3

9. The most important difference between infants and children and adults involves the *airway*. p. 458, Objective 2

10. B. The airway is smaller and therefore more easily blocked by fluid, secretions, or swelling. p. 458, Objectives 2, 4

11. D. The large tongue of a child takes up proportionally more room in the mouth and can cause airway compromise. p. 458, Objectives 2, 4

12. As children work hard to breathe, they will become *fatigued*. The increased work of breathing

uses a tremendous amount of energy, and muscles will tire. p. 458, Objective 2

13. To prevent occlusion, or kinking, of the airway, a head-tilt, chin-lift maneuver should put the head into a *neutral* position, in which the nose points straight up. p. 458, Objectives 2, 7

14. True. Do not insert the suction catheter further than you can see and be sure to measure the length of the catheter prior to insertion. p. 459, Objective 7

15. Suction should be limited to *10 to 15* seconds, and you should always apply *oxygen* before and after suctioning. p. 459, Objective 7

16. To insert an oropharyngeal airway in an infant or child, use a tongue depressor to push down the tongue and insert the airway without rotation. p. 459, Objective 7

17. Nasopharyngeal airways can be used when the patient has a *gag reflex*, whereas oropharyngeal airways cannot. p. 459, Objective 7

18. True. The oxygen is held close to the patient's face without placing a mask on the patient. Infants and children may tolerate this method of oxygen delivery better than a mask. p. 461, Objective 7

19. B. Adjust the flow rate to 5 L/min for infants and 10 L/min for children when applying blow-by oxygen. p. 461, Objective 7

20. B. Ventilate an infant or child every 3 seconds, or 20 times per minute. p. 462, Objective 7

21. Besides the gentle rise in the chest wall, other indicators of adequate ventilation in children are improvement in the *heart rate* and *skin color*. p. 462, Objective 2

22. With children, consider examining painful areas *last*. If the painful area is examined first, the child may be unwilling to allow you to complete your assessment. p. 463, Objectives 2, 3

23. The acronym AVPU stands for Alert, responsive to Verbal stimuli, responsive to Painful stimuli, and Unresponsive. p. 463

24. p—stridor on inspiration; l—expiratory wheeze; c—unable to cough or speak; l—skin may appear normal or cyanotic; c—skin may appear pale or cyanotic. p. 465, Objective 4

25. B. The care for responsive children with a foreign body airway obstruction is the same as for an adult. Unresponsive infants should receive back blows and chest thrusts but never abdominal thrusts. Blind finger sweeps should never be performed on infants—attempt to remove a foreign body only if you see the object. When performing abdominal thrusts on an unresponsive child, use the heel of one hand and perform up to five thrusts before inspecting the airway. p. 465, Objective 6

26. More than 80% of all cardiac arrests in children begin as *respiratory* arrests. Respiratory distress must be recognized early in children to prevent

further deterioration into cardiac arrest. p. 469, Objective 10

27. Signs of early respiratory distress in children include: increased rate of breathing; nasal flaring; intercostal and supraclavicular retractions; mottled skin color; use of abdominal muscles; see-saw respirations; stridor; wheezing; and grunting. p. 471, Objectives 4, 5

28. Signs of respiratory failure in children include: altered mental status; respiratory rate over 60 or under 20 breaths per minute with signs of fatigue; severe retractions; severe use of accessory muscles; decreased muscle tone; cyanosis; and poor peripheral perfusion. p. 472, Objectives 4, 5

29. A seizure can be caused by a rapid rise in a *fever*. Seizures also can be caused by chronic medical conditions, infection, poisoning, low blood sugar, head injury, hypoxia, and unknown causes. p. 472, Objective 11

30. C. A nasopharyngeal airway can be a useful adjunct to help control the patient's airway following a seizure. The recovery position should be used only if there is no known or suspected trauma to the head or spine. Do not put anything in the patient's mouth while the patient is having a seizure. Seizures are not always dangerous, but long (greater than 10 minutes) or repeated seizures may require the use of antiseizure medication. p. 473, Objective 12

31. Common signs and symptoms of shock in infants and children include: rapid respiratory rate; pale or mottled skin; cool, clammy skin; rapid pulse; weak or absent peripheral pulse; decreased blood pressure; absence of tears when crying; and poor urinary output and delayed capillary refill. p. 474, Objectives 8, 9

32. The top priority in the treatment of near-drowning cases is adequate *ventilation* and *oxygen*. p. 475

33. A. SIDS generally occurs in patients less than 1 year of age. Follow basic life-support procedures and transport the infant to the nearest appropriate facility. p. 475

34. Because it is larger and heavier than the other parts of the body, the *head* is the most frequently injured part of a child's body. p. 475, Objective 13

35. C. Hypothermia is a concern for any burned patient but especially children and the elderly. The skin has been injured and cannot regulate body temperature. p. 478, Objective 14

36. PASG may be indicated for children who have sustained trauma with signs and symptoms of hypoperfusion and pelvic instability. The PASG should not be used if there is evidence of penetrating chest trauma. Inflation of the abdominal compartment may hinder breathing and must be carefully monitored. Follow local protocol and advice

from medical direction regarding the use of PASG for pediatric patients. p. 478, Objective 14

37. Signs and symptoms of abuse include: multiple bruises in various stages of healing; injury inconsistent with the mechanism described by parent or caretaker; mechanism of injury inconsistent with child's developmental characteristics; repeated calls to the same address; fresh burns, especially on the feet, hands, and back; parents or caretakers who seem inappropriately unconcerned; conflicting histories given by parents or caretakers; and children afraid to discuss how the injury occurred. p. 479, Objective 15

38. True. When you treat an infant or child, you must also deal with the fears and concerns of the parent. p. 480

39. **a.** Has the child had previous seizures? Does the child take antiseizure medications? If she has had previous seizures, ask if this seizure was similar to others? p. 474. **b.** Common antiseizure medications include phenobarbital, Tegretol, Clonopin, depakene, and Dilantin. p. 474. **c.** Ensure a patent airway; have suction available; place the patient in the recovery position and monitor the airway; provide high-concentration oxygen; request advanced life-support resources if the seizure activity resumes; and transport per medical direction. p. 474

40. **a.** You suspect internal blood loss from an abdominal injury. p. 477. **b.** The decreased blood pressure and increased pulse and respiratory rates indicate that the patient's status may be deteriorating. These are signs of hypoperfusion. **c.** With any change in patient condition, contact medical direction and advise them of the change. You should apply continue high-concentration oxygen and repeat the ongoing assessment every 5 minutes. p. 483. **d.** Have suction available and turn the spine board on its side. p. 483

● **DIVISION SIX EXAMINATION**

1. A. Newborns and infants generally do not like to be separated from their parents, but they do not mind being assessed by strangers. EMT–Basics should assess the newborn in a way that prevents excessive heat loss. p. 456, Objective 1

2. D. Adolescents are not quite adults, but they should be treated as adults. Respect their right to modesty and privacy, and assess them apart from parents or other children. p. 458, Objective 1

3. A. Infants are obligate nose breathers, so the nostrils and nasopharynx should be suctioned if necessary to ease breathing. A child's tongue is relatively large in relationship to the mouth and often causes airway compromise. Children compensate for airway compromise by increasing their breathing rate and effort. An infant's airway is less developed and more flexible than an adult's. p. 458, Objective 2

4. C. Nasal airways are useful for maintaining an open airway when a patient's muscles relax following a seizure. The nasal airway can be inserted into either nostril, as long as it is inserted without force. Oral airways are more likely than nasal airways to stimulate vomiting. The preferred method for inserting an oral airway in a child patient is by using a tongue depressor. p. 459, Objective 7

5. B. Parents can be used to help deliver oxygen to pediatric patients; the children are more comfortable with their parents and the parent will feel useful. Blow-by oxygen means that the oxygen source is about 5 cm from the patient's face. Nonrebreather masks can be used for any patient who needs to receive high-concentration oxygen. The flow rate for a nonrebreather mask should be 12 to 15 L/min to ensure that enough oxygen is being delivered through the mask. p. 461, Objective 7

6. A. Ventilate the child until you see a gentle chest rise, rather than trying to determine the tidal volume required for each patient. The ventilation rate for children is one breath every 3 seconds, or 20 breaths per minute. The bag used should be at least 450 to 750 mL and should not have a pop-off valve to ensure adequate tidal volumes and ventilation pressure. p. 462, Objective 3

7. B. Mottled skin is an early finding of inadequate oxygenation in children, often seen before cyanosis. Children are considered to be responsive to verbal stimulus if they recognize their parent's voice, because children may be unable to understand and follow commands. Capillary refill should take less than 2 seconds in a patient who is perfusing adequately. When assessing a child, use the trunk-to-head approach to avoid scaring the child. p. 463, Objectives 7, 8

8. D. Assess the pulse of an infant at the femoral or brachial artery. Assess the pulse of children and adults at the radial or carotid artery. p. 464, Objective 9

9. C. Assess blood pressure for patients older than 3 years of age. p. 464, Objective 9

10. B. Abdominal thrusts alone are used for children and adults with a foreign body airway obstruction. Back blows and chest thrusts are used for infants with a foreign body airway obstruction. p. 469, Objective 6

11. A. Complete upper airway obstruction is characterized by: a sick general appearance; gasping or no respirations; pale to cyanotic skin color; inability to cough or speak; and a possible history of foreign body obstruction or cold symptoms. Partial upper airway obstruction is characterized by a relatively well to sick general appearance; increased work of breathing; normal to pale skin color;

inspiratory stridor or crowing; and a history suggestive of foreign body obstruction. Patients with lower airway disease exhibit signs and symptoms such as a relatively well to very sick appearance; increased work of breathing; normal to cyanotic skin color; expiratory wheezes; and a history of airway disease. p. 465, Objective 6

12. A. Wheezing is a sign of early respiratory distress, along with increased rate of breathing, nasal flaring, intercostal and supraclavicular retractions, mottled skin color, use of abdominal muscles, seesaw respirations, stridor, and grunting. Signs of respiratory failure include altered mental status, cyanosis, respiratory rate over 60 or under 20 breaths per minute, severe retractions, severe use of accessory muscles, decreased muscle tone, and poor peripheral perfusion. p. 472, Objective 5

13. C. Altered mental status may be caused by a diabetic emergency, poisoning, seizure, infection, head trauma, hypoxia, and shock. The EMT–Basic should care for the seizure patient without trying to diagnose the cause of the seizure. Airway and ventilation are the primary concern for the near-drowning patient. Activated charcoal can be administered to alert responsive children with the consent of medical direction. p. 473, Objective 12

14. D. SIDS deaths do not have a clear history or a factor that points to the cause of death. Patients who are abused may present to the EMT–Basic as a SIDS death. Do not question the parents at the scene but do note any signs of abuse or neglect and report them to the appropriate authorities. SIDS is most common in the first year of life. Unless the patient has rigor mortis, attempt to resuscitate the patient with good basic life-support skills. p. 475, Objective 15

15. B. Blunt trauma is most common in children, but penetrating trauma, burns, and immersion injuries are also common. p. 475, Objective 13

16. A. Because of its size and weight, the head is the most commonly injured area of a child. p. 477, Objective 13

17. C. In an unresponsive patient, the tongue commonly falls back into the airway causing obstruction. The jaw thrust maneuver should be used to open the airway without moving the patient's neck. p. 477, Objective 14

18. C. Signs of abuse and neglect include: multiple bruises in various stages of healing; injury inconsistent with the mechanism described by caretaker; mechanism of injury inconsistent with the child's developmental characteristics; repeated calls for the same child; fresh burns; parents who seem inappropriately unconcerned; conflicting histories given by parents; and the child being afraid to discuss the injury. Do not question the parents at the scene, but report suspicions to the appropriate authorities. Neglect is giving insufficient attention or respect to a child. Abuse occurs when actions harm a child. p. 479, Objectives 15, 16

19. C. The tube placed directly into the stomach to feed a patient is called a gastric tube. Tracheostomy tubes are used for breathing. Central lines provide venous access. p. 480

20. C. Parents are often anxious because they are worried about the health of their child and they feel helpless. Allow the parents to help care for the child when possible, and answer their questions honestly. p. 481

● CHAPTER 30
AMBULANCE OPERATIONS

● MATCHING
1. F
2. C
3. E
4. B
5. A
6. D

Definitions to key terms can be found on page 489 of the student textbook. Key terms cover Objectives 6 and 13.

● REVIEW QUESTIONS
1. Preparation for the call includes checking availability and readiness of *vehicle, medical supplies,* and *personnel.* p. 490, Objective 2

2. True. Continuing education keeps you up to date on current information and is considered preparation for the call and for treating patients. p. 490, Objective 2

3. Personal protective equipment includes gloves, mask, goggles or other eye protection, and gown. p. 491

4. True. Nonmedical equipment should be stocked and checked at the beginning of every ambulance shift just as you would for medical equipment. Nonmedical equipment includes personal protective equipment, maps, reference books, etc. p. 491, Objective 1

5. True. Different systems give you different dispatch information, but you will generally receive information about the location and nature of illness/ mechanism of injury, number of patients, severity of injuries or illness, patient age, and scene hazards. p. 492, Objective 7

6. D. Safe drivers are physically and mentally fit, are able to perform under stress, have a positive attitude, and are tolerant of other drivers, in addition to the items listed in the question. p. 493, Objective 4

7. False. Drivers are sometimes startled when they see an emergency vehicle and may drive erratically. p. 493, Objective 4

8. Factors contributing to emergency vehicle crashes include: excessive speed; reckless driving; failing to obey traffic signals or posted speed limits; disregarding traffic rules and regulations; failing to heed traffic warning signals; inadequate dispatch information; escorts; multiple-vehicle response; and failure to anticipate the actions of other drivers. p. 494, Objectives 4, 5

9. E. During the time while en route to the scene, get more information from dispatch if it is available and plan for the equipment and personnel you may need on the scene. p. 494, Objective 2

10. The first priority in parking at the scene is *safety*. p. 494, Objective 2

11. C. When you arrive at the scene, begin the scene size-up and call for additional resources as necessary. p. 495, Objective 2

12. False. You should only drive with lights and sirens to the hospital when the patient condition warrants it. Not every response is an emergency, and it is not worth the risk of a traffic accident to respond with lights and siren to a nonemergency. p. 495, Objective 8

13. C. While en route to the receiving facility, complete the detailed physical examination (if necessary) and perform ongoing assessments based on the patient's condition. The initial assessment and focused history and physical examination should occur on scene before the patient is moved. Life-threatening injuries should be treated as soon as they are found. p. 495, Objective 2

14. Patient transfer includes putting the patient in the appropriate room and giving the *patient* report. p. 495, Objective 2

15. False. Documentation should be completed before leaving the receiving facility so that your prehospital care report will be available if the staff has any questions and so it can become part of the patient's permanent record. p. 495, Objective 10

16. C. Low-level disinfection is used for routine cleaning when no body fluids are present. p. 496, Objective 14

17. A. High-level disinfection is used for equipment that is involved in invasive procedures. p. 496, Objective 14

18. Restocking and rechecking inventory occurs during the *postrun* phase. p. 497, Objectives 11, 12

19. Mechanism of injury situations for possible air medical transport include: vehicle rollover in which there are unrestrained passengers; pedestrian struck by a car at speeds greater than 10 mph; a fall of greater than 15 ft; motorcycle crashes at greater than 10 mph; collision involving death of other occupants of same vehicle; and ejection from a vehicle. p. 498

20. True. The pilot needs to know that you are near the aircraft to avoid injury. p. 500

21. **a.** When called to the scene of a cardiac emergency, you should take basic supplies, patient transfer equipment, suction equipment, artificial ventilation devices, oxygen administration equipment, cardiac compression equipment, and AED. p. 491. **b.** Due regard for others includes: adequate notice of approach to prevent a collision and understanding and following state laws and regulations regarding vehicle stopping, procedures at red lights, stop signs, and intersections, speed limits, direction of traffic flow, and specified turns. p. 494. **c.** When you arrive at the receiving facility, be sure to: notify dispatch; transfer the patient to the appropriate room; provide a brief report that contains all pertinent information to the receiving staff; restock the ambulance and complete the prehospital care report to be left with the patient's chart; and wash your hands and perform infection control measures as necessary. p. 495

● CHAPTER 31
GAINING ACCESS

● REVIEW QUESTIONS

1. Extrication is the process of removing a patient from entanglement in a motor vehicle or other situation in a safe and appropriate manner. p. 506, Objective 1

2. The role of the incident commander is to *coordinate* efforts of medical and rescue personnel. p. 506, Objective 4

3. True. Not all extrication will require special equipment to remove the patient, but special protective equipment and knowledge is always needed. p. 506, Objective 3

4. In all cases of entrapment, *critical patient care* precedes extrication. p. 507, Objective 2

5. A. EMS and rescue personnel should work together to coordinate the safest and most efficient way to remove a patient. EMS personnel are responsible for patient care and critical interventions. p. 508, Objective 2

6. At the scene the EMT should be concerned with: 1) personal safety, then 2) safety of the crew, 3) safety of the patient, and 4) bystander safety. p. 508, Objective 2

7. Protective gear during a rescue operation should include: impact-resistant protective helmet with ear protection and chin strap; protective eyewear; turn-out coat; leather gloves; and boots with steel insole and toes. p. 508, Objective 3

8. B. Patients are covered during an extrication to protect them from flying debris. A blanket also

may be necessary to keep the patient warm. p. 508, Objective 5

9. False. Every extrication has potential for hazards. Bystanders will be at potential risk and should be kept clear of the area. p. 509, Objective 2

10. Potential hazards at the scene of an automobile crash include: hazardous materials; fire; electrical wires; and unstable vehicles.

11. The safety officer is an *objective* observer who helps identify additional *hazards* not readily apparent to the rescuers. p. 510, Objective 4

12. Simple access does not require the use of rescue equipment to access the patient. Complex access required additional education, skills, and rescue equipment. p. 511, Objectives 6, 7

13. There are many types of specialized rescues including: vehicle rescue; water rescue; trench rescue; and high-angle rescue. p. 511

14. B. The patient can be moved if he/she is in danger or cannot be treated in the position he/she is in. EMT–Basics must immobilize the patient prior to transport even if the patient has no pain or other complaints. p. 511, Objective 6

15. False. Two people will not be enough to safely move the patient and maintain spinal alignment. Three or four people are recommended. p. 511

16. **a.** Personal safety is the first priority followed by the safety of your crew, the patients, and bystanders. p. 508. **b.** Personal protective equipment for this scene includes impact-resistant protective helmet with ear protection and chin strap; protective eyewear; puncture-resistant "turn-out" coat; leather gloves; and boots with steel insoles and steel toes. p. 508. **c.** Only utility or rescue workers educated in managing live power lines should approach the lines or secure them. Advise the victims to stay inside the wreckage. Talk to them through a loud speaker or public address system. Have the appropriate agency respond to the scene. You cannot make the scene safe, so do not enter. p. 509

● CHAPTER 32
OVERVIEWS: SPECIAL
RESPONSE SITUATIONS

● MATCHING

1. B
2. H
3. E
4. K
5. A
6. C
7. F
8. D
9. J
10. I
11. G

Definitions to key terms can be found on page 515 of the student textbook.

● REVIEW QUESTIONS

1. False. Although there are large supplies of hazardous materials at most industrial sites, a hazardous materials incident can occur on the street, at a public pool or school, or at home. p. 516

2. The primary concern at any hazardous material scene is *safety*. p. 517, Objective 1

3. Always approach a hazardous material scene from an *uphill* and *upwind* direction. p. 518, Objective 5

4. C. The size and shape of a container may give you an idea of the contents. p. 518

5. True. As always, if the scene is unsafe and you can not make it safe, do not enter. p. 518, Objectives 2, 5

6. A. Every EMT should be educated to at least the *First Responder Awareness* level of hazardous materials knowledge. p. 516, Objective 1

7. When approaching a potential hazardous materials situation: a) approach from an uphill and upwind direction; b) isolate the area; c) avoid contact with the area; d) be alert for unusual odors, clouds, and leakage; e) remember that some chemicals are odorless; f) do not drive through leakage or vapor clouds; g) keep all personnel and bystanders a safe distance from the scene; h) approach the scene with extreme caution. p. 518, Objectives 3, 5

8. Sources of information and assistance for hazardous materials can be found on placards, MSDS, Emergency Response Guidebook, and CHEMTREC. p. 519, Objectives 4, 5

9. Incident management systems: a) provide a group leader; b) provide for orderly communications; d) provide for interactions between many agencies; and e) help with decision making. Management systems cannot supply unlimited resources. p. 521, Objective 11

10. A major incident should be declared when: 1) the situation requires great demand on resources, equipment, or personnel; 2) any hazardous materials situation; 3) any situation requiring special resources; 4) anytime you are unsure if an incident management system is needed p. 521, Objective 7

11. The *treatment* sector provides care for patients as they are received from triage and extrication. p. 522, Objective 11

12. The *supply* sector provides resources, supplies, personnel, and equipment. p. 522, Objective 11

13. Within each sector there is a *sector officer* who runs the operation of the sector. p. 522, Objective 11

14. D. If the incident command system is already established when the EMT–Basic arrives on scene, report to the staging area for an assignment. Report to the

sector officer to whom you are assigned and ask for specific instructions. p. 523, Objectives 8, 10

15. A method of categorizing patient treatment and transport needs is called *triage*. p. 522, Objective 9

16. Triage tags are used to identify the needs of large numbers of patients, so that other members of the team can quickly identify their illness/injury without completing an assessment. p. 523, Objective 9

17. a—severed artery in leg; c—contusion and laceration to forearm; a—circumferential burn to chest; c—absent pulse and respirations; c—deformity to one wrist with contusions; a—burns to arms, hands, and feet; a—cool, clammy skin, low blood pressure, rapid heart rate; b—pain, swelling, and deformity to thigh; b—severe back and neck pain, motor, sensory functions intact. p. 524, Objective 9

18. **a.** Major incidents include: situations requiring a great demand on resources, equipment, or personnel; any hazardous materials situation; any situation requiring special fire, rescue, law enforcement, or EMS resources; and any situation in which you are unsure whether the incident management system is needed. p. 521. **b.** EMS sectors include incident command; extrication; treatment; transportation; staging; supply; and triage. p. 522. **c.** As triage officer, you should move rapidly through the patients, doing an initial assessment and using triage tags to assign patients in treatment categories. As patients are assessed and tagged, they are moved to a treatment area for further evaluation and intervention. p. 524

● DIVISION SEVEN EXAMINATION

1. B. Splinting supplies are the only basic equipment listed. Advanced supplies may be used by EMT-Intermediates or –Paramedics who are educated for advanced procedures. EMT–Basics should have basic supplies, patient transfer equipment, airway and ventilation equipment, wound care supplies, splinting material, an OB kit, medications (oxygen, activated charcoal, and glucose), and an AED. p. 491, Objective 1

2. A. When en route to an emergency call, be sure to use safety belts, drive carefully, obey traffic laws, and have due regard for others. Red lights and sirens should be used for true emergencies. Discuss equipment that may be needed for this call and obtain additional information if it is available. p. 494, Objectives 2, 6

3. D. When parking at the scene of an emergency, park uphill and upwind from any hazardous material, position the unit for departure from the scene, park at least 30 m from any wreckage, and use emergency lights to notify others of your presence. p. 495, Objective 3

4. D. When arriving at the scene, notify dispatch and record the time of arrival, perform the scene size-up, and call for additional help if necessary. p. 495, Objective 3

5. B. Perform ongoing assessments while en route to the receiving facility. Care for life-threatening injuries should be provided immediately when the life threat is found. The initial assessment should be performed when you first arrive at the patient's side. Billing and insurance information can be obtained at the receiving facility. p. 495, Objective 2

6. B. Give a radio report to the receiving facility staff while en route to the facility to alert them about the patient's condition. Another report should be given at bedside. p. 495, Objective 2

7. C. Airway equipment and other pieces of equipment that come in contact with mucous membranes require high-level disinfection. Dressings should be disposable and used for only one patient. Items such as blood pressure cuffs and penlights can be cleaned, or they may be disposable. p. 497, Objective 13

8. A. Landing zones for EMS helicopters ideally should be 30 m by 30 m, and minimally 18 m by 18 m. p. 499

9. C. The decision to use an EMS helicopter is based on time and distance considerations and illness and injury considerations. Helicopters can be used for critically ill patients, as well as for injured patients. For safety, approach the helicopter from the front so the pilot can see you and from the downhill side for maximum clearance of the rotor blades. p. 500

10. C. Personal protective equipment such as gloves, boots, eye protection, turnout coats, and helmets should be worn for every rescue situation. Simple access means no special tools are required to extricate the patient. Personal safety is always the priority, followed by safety of other crew members, the patient, and bystanders. Patients should be immobilized if the mechanism of injury suggests spinal trauma, whether the patient has pain or not. p. 511, Objectives 3, 5, 7

11. D. EMT–Basics not involved in rescue should work with rescue workers while providing emergency care for the patient and protecting them from further injury. p. 508, Objective 2

12. D. Chemtrec provides a 24-hour hotline for information about chemicals and advice for emergency personnel working at hazardous materials scenes. p. 520

13. B. EMT–Basics should be educated to at least the first responder awareness level for hazardous materials. This level is designed for those individuals who are likely to discover a hazardous materials incident. p. 520, Objective 1

14. B. Park the ambulance uphill and upwind from hazardous materials. Hazardous materials are

found in the home, office, recreational areas, and in industry. Some chemicals are odorless and colorless, so do not enter the scene until someone with the appropriate education determines that the scene is safe. p. 528, Objective 4

15. A. The transportation sector coordinates ambulance, hospital, and air medical resources. The staging sector coordinates movement of vehicles from the scene. The support sector or supply sector obtains resources and supplies. p. 522, Objective 11

16. C. Triage means categorizing patients based on the severity of their illness or injury, so that the most critical patients will be treated and transported first. p. 523, Objective 9

17. D. EMT–Basics should categorize patients based on severity of injury or illness and correct only life-threatening injuries during triage. p. 523, Objective 9

18. D. Patients with no pulse or respirations are considered to be the lowest priority. p. 524, Objective 9

19. A. Patients with airway or breathing difficulties, uncontrolled or severe bleeding, decreased or altered mental status, severe medical problems, signs and symptoms of shock, and severe burns with respiratory compromise are considered to be priority patients. p. 523, Objective 9

● CHAPTER 33
ADVANCED AIRWAY TECHNIQUES

● MATCHING

1. O
2. D
3. M
4. L
5. I
6. A
7. F
8. T
9. B
10. U
11. H
12. R
13. G
14. P
15. J
16. K
17. E
18. N
19. Q
20. C
21. S

Definitions to key terms can be found on page 531 of the student textbook.

● REVIEW QUESTIONS

1. The Sellick maneuver is designed to reduce gastric distention during artificial ventilation. The Sellick maneuver will also help prevent passive regurgitation during artificial ventilation. p. 533, Objective 7

2. B. The cricoid ring is inferior to the cricothyroid membrane and is the location where pressure is applied during the Sellick maneuver. p. 533, Objectives 1, 7

3. True. Releasing the Sellick maneuver may cause the patient to vomit. The maneuver must be maintained until an endotracheal tube is inserted and the position of the tube is confirmed. p. 533, Objective 7

4. Indications for adult endotracheal intubation include: when you cannot ventilate an apneic patient; when the patient is unresponsive; when a patient has no gag reflex or coughing; or when a patient cannot protect the airway. p. 534, Objective 8

5. **a.** Open end; **b.** 15-mm adapter; **c.** Pilot balloon; **d.** Inflation valve; **e.** Syringe; **f.** Open end; **g.** Murphy's eye; **h.** Inflatable cuff. p. 535, Objective 9

6. B. Although you should evaluate every patient individually, most men will require an 8- to 8.5-mm internal diameter tube; most women will require a 7- to 8-mm internal diameter tube. In an emergency, a 7.5-mm tube will work for almost any adult patient. p. 537, Objective 13

7. A stylet is inserted into the tube to make it stiff and help it maintain shape during the intubation procedure. The pilot balloon indicates whether the cuff at the distal end of the tube has been inflated—if the pilot balloon is inflated, the cuff is inflated. Murphy's eye is an opening at the end of the endotracheal tube that decreases the chance of obstruction if the tip of the tube is blocked. p. 537, Objective 12

8. The straight, or Miller blade, lifts the epiglottis directly, allowing the EMT–Basic to visualize the vocal cords. The tip of the curved, or MacIntosh, blade is inserted into the vallecula and lifts just in front of the epiglottis to help visualize the cords. p. 537, Objectives 10, 11

9. False. Tape can be used to secure the tube in place, or a commercial device may be used. Discuss the methods for securing an endotracheal tube in place with your medical director and be sure to know what methods are approved in your region. A bite block should also be inserted to prevent the patient from biting on the tube. p. 537, Objective 21

10. C. The infant patient may require padding to be placed under the upper back to elevate the shoulders. This will help bring the structures of the air-

way into alignment for intubation. The adult patient's head should be placed in a sniffing position before intubation. The endotracheal tube should be inserted until the cuff just passes the vocal cords (Murphy's eye is distal to the cuff on the endotracheal tube). The Sellick maneuver should be performed on all patients prior to intubation to decrease the risks of gastric distention and vomiting. p. 538, 548, Objectives 17, 18

11. C. When there are gurgling sounds in the stomach during ventilation, the endotracheal tube is most likely in the esophagus and should be removed immediately. Esophageal intubation means that the patient is receiving no oxygen when ventilated. p. 540, Objectives 19, 20

12. B. When there are breath sounds only on the right side following intubation, the tube is most likely in the right mainstem bronchus. Deflate the cuff with the syringe and pull the tube back until breath sounds are equal bilaterally. Reinflate the cuff and secure the tube in place. p. 540, Objective 19

13. C. No more than 30 seconds should elapse between the time the last ventilation is delivered and when the next ventilation is delivered through the endotracheal tube. If the intubation procedure cannot be completed in 30 seconds, ventilate the patient with high-flow oxygen before attempting to intubate. p. 541, Objective 17

14. Complications of intubation include: esophageal intubation; chipped teeth and trauma to soft tissue; decreased heart rate; hypoxia; mainstem intubation; vomiting; and self-extubation. p. 542, Objective 15

15. The two indications for tracheal suctioning for the EMT–Basic are secretions seen coming out of the endotracheal tube and poor compliance when ventilating. p. 542

16. D. Nasogastric tubes are indicated for patients who cannot be ventilated because of gastric distention. A nasogastric tube will relieve the pressure, making ventilation more successful. p. 543, Objective 6

17. C. The cricoid ring is the narrowest portion of the airway in infants and children, which is why endotracheal tubes are not cuffed for this age group. The airway structures of pediatric patients are softer and more flexible than adults. The tongue is larger and takes up more space proportionally in the mouth than in adults. The trachea and vocal cords of children are higher and lie more anteriorly than in adults. p. 545, Objectives 1, 2

18. Infants and children should be intubated when: prolonged artificial ventilation is needed, making gastric distention likely; artificial ventilation cannot be achieved by any other method; the patient is apneic; or the patient is unresponsive, without a cough or a gag reflex. p. 545, Objective 18

19. A. The formula, (16 + age in years) divided by 4, is an excellent guide for endotracheal tube selection in children. The child must be over 2 years of age, and the age used in the formula must be in years, not months. p. 546, Objective 14

20. A child's airway size can be approximated by using the size of the little finger and the inside diameter of the nostril. There also are formulas and charts to help determine the correct size for airway equipment. Be sure to have a tube 0.5 mm smaller and larger than the estimated correct tube size. p. 546, Objective 16

21. False. A slow heart rate in a child is a sign of hypoxia. p. 549, Objective 18

22. B. The risk of a mainstem intubation is greater in infants and children, due to the short distance from the vocal cords to the carina. p. 549, Objective 18

23. a. Endotracheal intubation is the most effective way to manage a patient's airway and is the best way to ventilate an apneic patient who has no gag reflex. Endotracheal intubation minimizes the risk of aspiration and allows for better oxygen delivery to the lungs; provides complete control of the airway; and allows for suctioning of the trachea and bronchi. p. 534. b. When performing endotracheal intubation, you will need a laryngoscope handle; curved and straight blades; Magill forceps; endotracheal tube; stylet; lubrication; OP airway; and tape. p. 537. c. The tube most likely has been inserted too far and has come to rest in the right mainstem bronchi. You should deflate the cuff and slowly withdraw the tube while continuing to ventilate until you hear breath sounds. Ensure that right and left chest sounds are equal and reinflate the cuff. p. 540

● DIVISION EIGHT EXAMINATION

1. A. The Sellick maneuver is used to prevent passive regurgitation when a patient cannot protect his/her own airway. The maneuver also reduces gastric distention. p. 533, Objective 7

2. B. The cricoid ring is inferior to the cricothyroid membrane. To locate the cricoid ring, find the thyroid cartilage and the depression just below it (the cricothyroid membrane). The cricoid ring is just below the cricothyroid membrane. p. 533, Objective 7

3. D. EMT–Basics use orotracheal intubation techniques, which means that the endotracheal tube is passed through the patient's mouth and into the trachea. p. 534, Objective 17

4. C. EMT–Basics should intubate apneic patients who cannot be ventilated and patients who are unresponsive to any painful stimuli and have no gag reflex. EMT–Basics should also intubate any patient who cannot protect his/her own airway for any reason. p. 534, Objective 8

5. B. A 7.5-mm i.d. endotracheal tube will work for most patients in an emergency setting. Adult men usually require a 8.0 to 8.5-mm i.d. tube, and adult women usually require a 7.0 to 8.0-mm i.d. endotracheal tube. p. 537, Objective 13

6. C. The tip of the curved blade is placed into the vallecula, the anatomic space between the base of the tongue and the epiglottis. When the blade is lifted, the epiglottis is lifted also. The tip of the straight blade is used to lift the epiglottis out of the way to allow you to visualize the vocal cords. p. 537, Objectives 10, 11

7. C. A water-soluble lubricant should be used to lubricate the distal end of the endotracheal tube so that it will slide easily into the trachea. The stylet also can be lubricated if necessary so that it will slide into and out of the endotracheal tube easily. p. 538, Objective 17

8. B. The tip of the stylet should be approximately 0.25 inches from the distal end of the cuff or the proximal end of Murphy's eye. This will prevent the tip of the stylet from extending beyond the endotracheal tube and causing damage to the patient's airway structures. p. 538, Objective 12

9. A. The laryngoscope handle is held in the left hand. The laryngoscope blade is inserted into the right side of the patient's mouth, and the tongue is swept to the left and out of the line of sight. p. 538, Objective 17

10. B. 5 to 10 cc of air should be inserted into the cuff. The air is injected through an inflation valve that also inflates the pilot balloon. The pilot balloon serves as a reminder if the cuff is inflated or not. p. 539, Objective 17

11. D. After intubation, auscultate over the epigastrium first. If you hear gurgling noises, the endotracheal tube is in the esophagus and should be removed immediately. p. 539, Objective 19

12. C. If gurgling is heard over the epigastrium, the tube is in the esophagus and should be removed immediately. When the endotracheal tube is in the esophagus, the patient is not being ventilated. Ventilate the patient for 2 to 5 minutes after removing the tube and then intubate again if indicated. p. 540, Objective 20

13. A. If the endotracheal tube is in the mainstem bronchus, the EMT–Basic will hear breath sounds over only one side of the chest. The cuff of the tube should be deflated, and the tube should be pulled back while the EMT–Basic listens to breath sounds. When breath sounds are heard equally over both sides, the cuff should be reinflated and the tube secured in place. p. 540, Objective 19

14. C. The cuff of a properly placed endotracheal tube should lie just beyond the vocal cords. The EMT–Basic should watch the tube pass through the vocal cords while intubating. p. 540, Objectives 17, 19

15. D. Complications of intubation include esophageal intubation, trauma to soft tissue and teeth, decreased heart rate, hypoxia, main-stem intubation, vomiting, and self-extubation. The alveoli are the small air sacs in the lungs where oxygenation occurs. p. 542, Objective 15

16. D. When suctioning the nasopharynx or inside the endotracheal tube, a soft catheter should be used. For tracheal suctioning, insert the suction catheter about 25 cm and withdraw in a twisting motion while applying suction. p. 542

17. C. A nasogastric tube is inserted into the stomach through the nose and the esophagus. The stomach then can be decompressed for easier ventilation. The nasogastric tube also can be used for gastric lavage, administering medications or nutrition, and diagnosing trauma patients in the hospital setting. An endotracheal tube is used for ventilation; a foley catheter is used for urinary bladder catheterization. p. 543, Objective 6

18. C. The straight blade, or Miller blade, is preferred when intubating pediatric patients because it provides for greater displacement of the tongue when visualizing the vocal cords. Children have proportionally larger tongues than adults, and this can make intubation difficult if not controlled properly by the blade. p. 545, Objective 18

19. A. To determine the appropriate size endotracheal tube for a pediatric patient older than 2 years of age, add 16 to the age in years and divide by 4. The size also can be estimated by comparing the tube with the size of the patient's little finger or the inside diameter of the nostril. p. 546, Objective 14

20. B. Pediatric endotracheal tubes generally have one or more black rings that serve as vocal cord markers. The markers help ensure that the tip of the tube is placed halfway between the vocal cords and the carina. Pediatric endotracheal tubes are also uncuffed, because the narrow cricoid ring provides a seal for the tube. p. 546, Objective 18